I0408721

Cartoons by Robin Crossman

Photographs by Vanessa Guillen

Copyright © 2018 by Rachel Donen

This book is not intended to be a substitute for the medical advice of a licensed physician. The reader should consult with a physician in matters relating to his/her health and particularly with respect to any symptoms that may require diagnosis or medical attention.

ISBN-13: 978-1545148938

ISBN-10: 1545148937

4-WEEK PROGRAM FOR PAIN THAT WON'T GO AWAY

BACK PAIN AGAIN?

by Rachel Donen

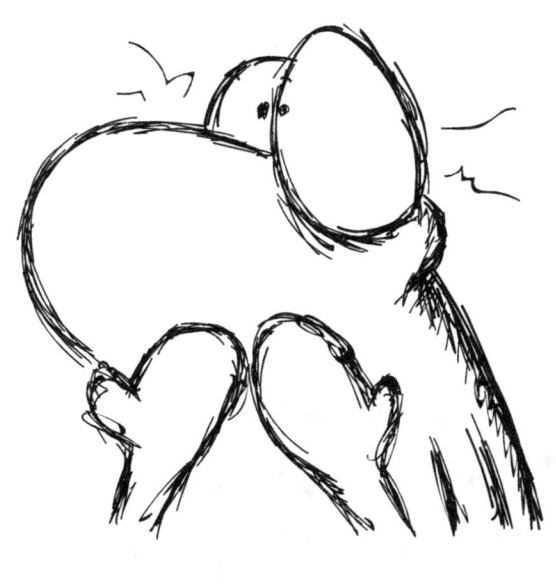

"If I'm this bad now, what's going to happen when I get older?"

"My back is aching again. What did I do wrong this time? Was it the way I moved? Did I do too much?"

"My back goes out every couple of months. What if I need surgery?"

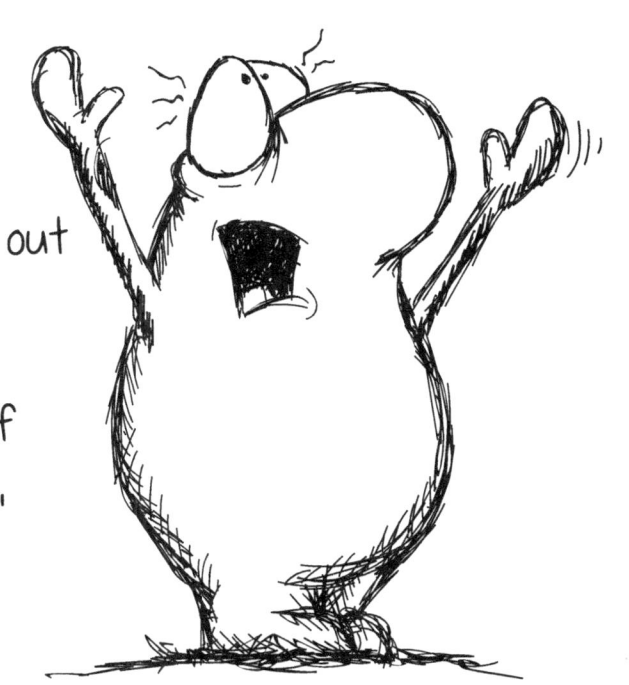

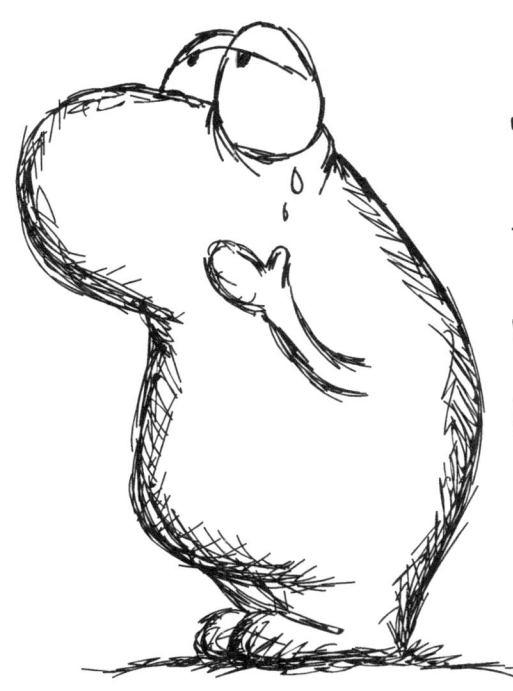

"How am I going to get better when exercise keeps hurting me."

Pain is exhausting and frustrating...

...especially when we've been doing physio, massage, seen our doctor... (add your list), but we just aren't getting better.

We want to be free to do the things we love again. We don't want to worry about the pain anymore.

This book is for all of the people still in pain who want to relieve pain, regain trust in their body, and get back to the things they love.

This book is Week 1, in a 4-week program to relieve pain.

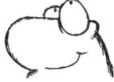

Contents

CHAPTER 1

Dissolving the worry about pain

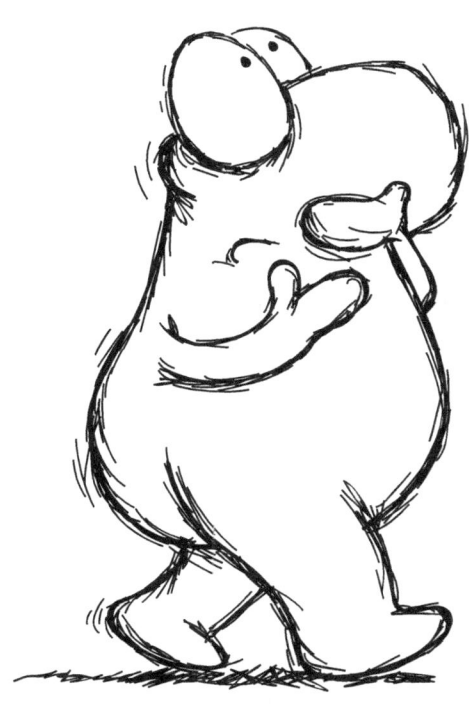

Worrying that something is wrong or...

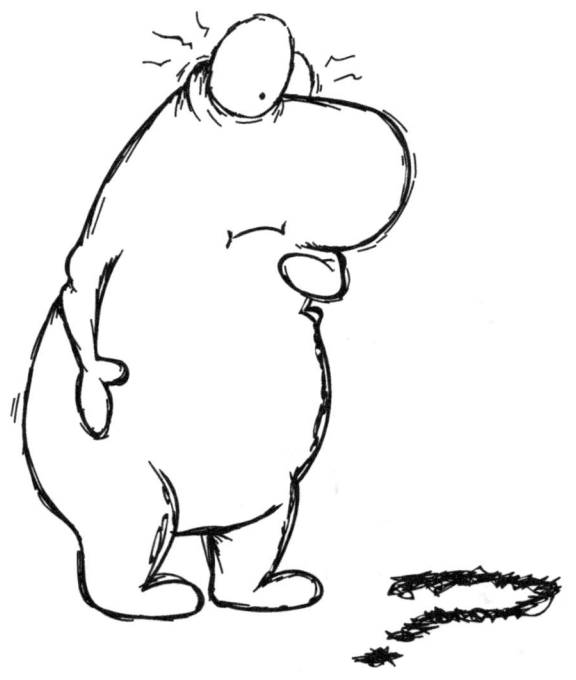

confusion about why we are still in
pain, will likely come up when we've
had pain over and over again.

To dissolve the worry and find peace,
we must first understand pain.

1. Pain does not always = damage

Damage does not always = pain

Especially with chronic pain
(pain that has been going on for three
months or longer)

Note. The term "damage" can be misused in the case of chronic pain when describing disc herniation, degeneration, and osteoarthritis. With aging, these are normal changes that can occur that the body can adapt to.

For many of my clients with chronic back pain, there is nothing structurally wrong. No injury. Or the injury they once had is healed but they still continue to have pain. And, for most of my other clients with chronic back pain, their pain is not related to things like their disc degeneration or herniated disc. This is good news, because this means:

→ There is no reason why they can't make a full recovery from chronic pain.

Usually this message of "there's nothing structurally wrong", or "their pain is not related to the disc degeneration or herniated disc that happened months or years ago", is difficult for new clients to hear...

"How could this be? I have pain all the time... and its been going on for a long time. Sometimes I can't even move. There must be something wrong? This must mean I'm still injured or else why would I have pain?... Right?"

Pain happens when we perceive we are in danger of an injury (whether there is damage or not).

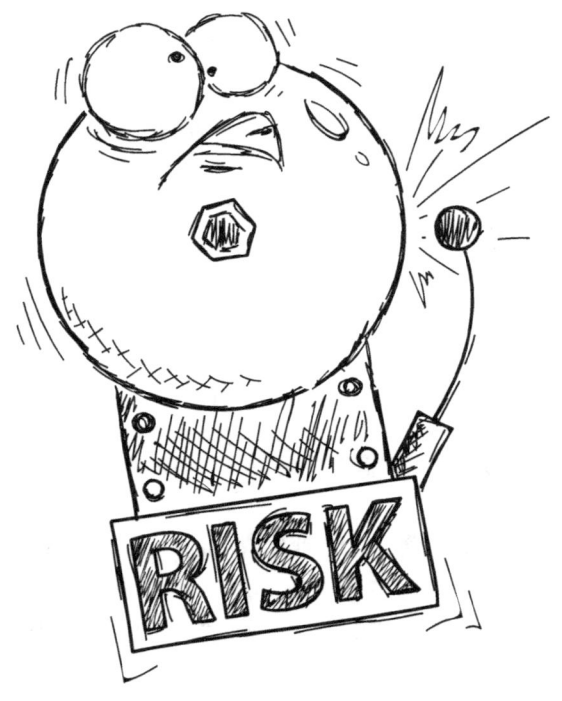

Once the brain thinks we are under threat, our nervous system goes on high alert to get the body into action to help out... to protect.

This type of description of pain was developed from studies in pain and neuroscience. See the book "Explain Pain" by Dr. David S. Butler and Prof. G. Lorimer Moseley for study references.

Note. The pain we experience is always real. What has changed is our understanding of what pain means and how it happens. Traditionally, we were taught that pain happens when the body picks up that there is damage, injury, or when something with the structure of the body is being hurt. Now we know that pain can happen without damage, injury, or the structure of the body being hurt; especially in the case of chronic pain. It is the perception that we are in danger, by our brain, that sets off the pain cycle.

This perception that we are in danger is formed when we interpret that the majority of information we hear, see, and feel says we are in danger of an injury...

says something bad is happening... says something's wrong.

Danger/Bad Info

"My bad side feels different from the other side. It feels weaker, stiff, less coordinated, it always hurts. There must be something wrong."

"I can't bend forward. I will hurt myself again."

"I feel exhausted."

"I must have moved the wrong way or done too much the other day."

Note. I have written the danger info as thoughts, because it's easier to understand this way. Some danger info starts as thoughts in the brain, but some start outside, like sensations from the muscles, increased amounts of stress hormones that keep being put into the body, and temperature changes indicating danger that we must then interpret.

We have just a moment to analyze all of this info (subconsciously or consciously) to see if we perceive we are in danger... to see if something bad is happening. And if it is, to determine how much, how bad, and what response.

This happens very quickly. We may not even know we are doing it.

As the danger info stacks up...

And the safe info is non-existent or much less...

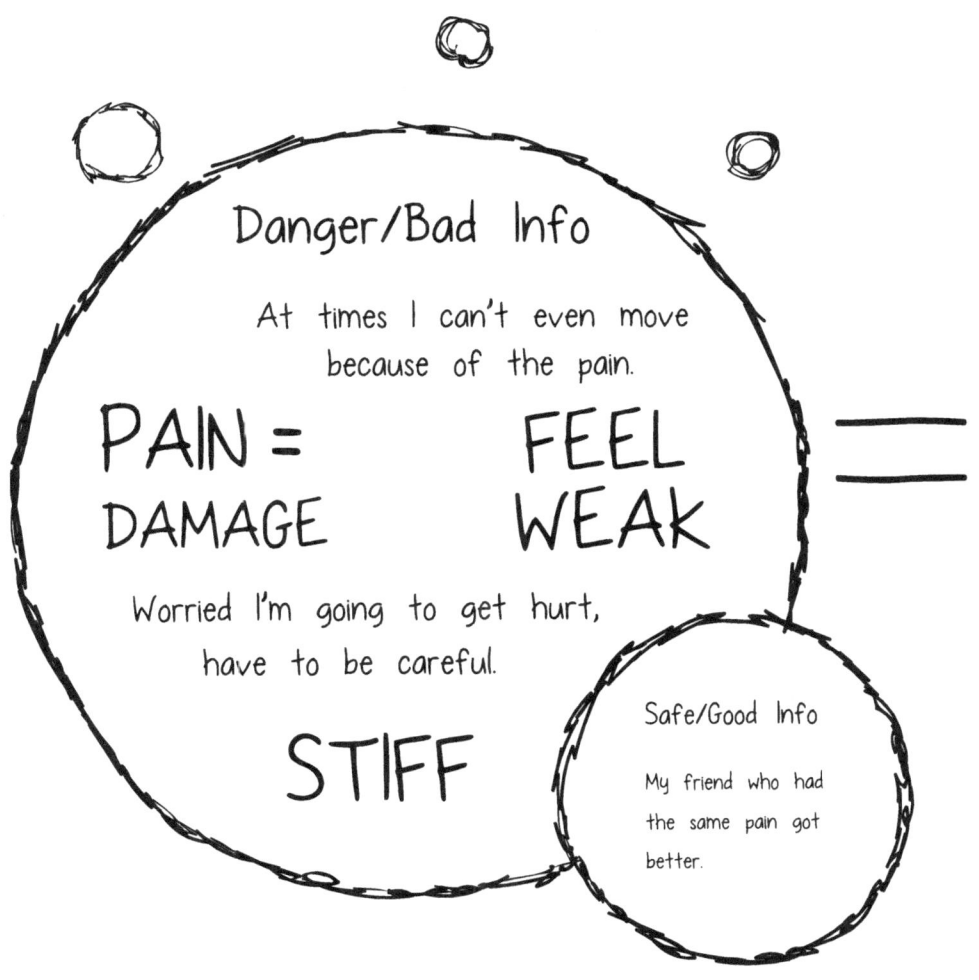

Danger/Bad Info

At times I can't even move because of the pain.

PAIN = DAMAGE

FEEL WEAK

Worried I'm going to get hurt, have to be careful.

STIFF

Safe/Good Info

My friend who had the same pain got better.

This overwhelming amount of bad info will tip us over to perceiving we are in danger, perceiving something bad is going to happen, perceiving something's wrong, perceiving we need to protect.

This is when pain happens.

Perception

$\longrightarrow$ "Something's wrong.
I'm vulnerable.
I need to protect."

2. Chronic pain changes our alarm system

If we believe that we are not safe, that we are damaged, that we will always have pain, and are in danger of hurting ourselves again... and again... and again; over time our nervous system's alarm bells will get louder... and louder... and louder. And be more easily set off. It becomes much easier to experience pain with this heightened sensitivity to any little cue we perceive is saying something bad is happening or is going to happen.

It's like if we walked through a dark alley over and over again, and every time, we thought we would be confronted by some creepy, menacing person yelling at us. We would feel unsafe each day; we would constantly feel we needed to protect ourselves. Any little sound or movement would make us flinch to protect.

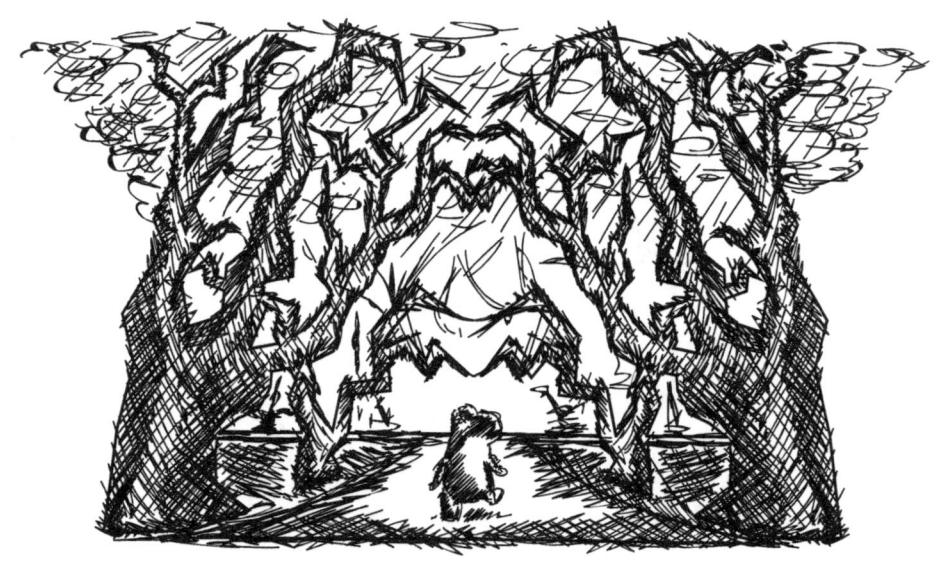

Our alarm system actually changes to become more sensitive to any possibility of danger (no matter how small) when we feel we are constantly under threat. Changes occur to our brain, neurons of the nervous system, and hormones released (e.g. more adrenaline to really get us worried).

Because of these changes, we become overly sensitive to any little possibility of danger and begin to send faulty danger alarms. And we tend not to catch the information that says we are o.k.... or we catch less of it... which can all lead to faulty interpretations of danger... something's wrong.

What we may not know is that we are referencing only from one particular story, "something's wrong". We have created a belief that we are vulnerable. That we need to protect that person who is vulnerable. We may not know that some, or all, of that story/belief may not be true anymore. And we may not know that we have a choice to reference something different.

We just need the opportunity to learn how to reference something new.... something that brings the feeling of safety... something that lets us see again how capable, strong, peaceful, and resilient we are. We do this so we can reverse the changes in our alarm system that has made it faulty.

So how do we do this?

What we need to do is calm those alarm bells.

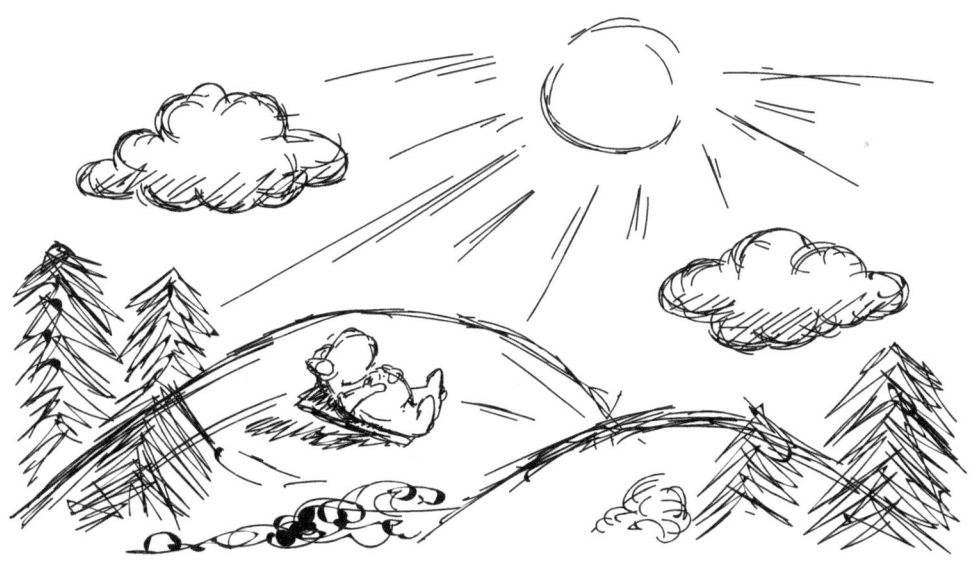

We do this by first re-discovering our sense of safety through knowledge of pain and direct experience/ practice of knowing when we are actually in danger of hurting ourselves and when we are not. The physical training will help us feel again how powerful, capable, and skilled our body is at this moment; and that our body can be a source of ease and comfort... further re-enforcing we are o.k. We don't need to protect.

The first focus of our physical and mental training for chronic pain must be to calm the alarm bells that say we are in danger and need to protect... when we are not actually in danger.

We do this by dissolving the protective patterns in the...

...Body

(tucking, holding, not moving, etc.)

...And Mind

(like worrying, monitoring for things that will hurt us, fear, etc.)

And also by re-discovering information, thoughts, sensations, movements, emotions, and experiences that let us know we are o.k.

So, when it comes time to look at all of the info to determine if we are in danger, more and more of it will be saying we are o.k.

Safe/Good Info

"I'm not broken... that makes me feel positive and hopeful."

"I feel strong."

"There is no reason why I can't recover from chronic pain."

"Feeling stiff, misaligned, and hearing my joints crack doesn't mean something's wrong. Who knew?"

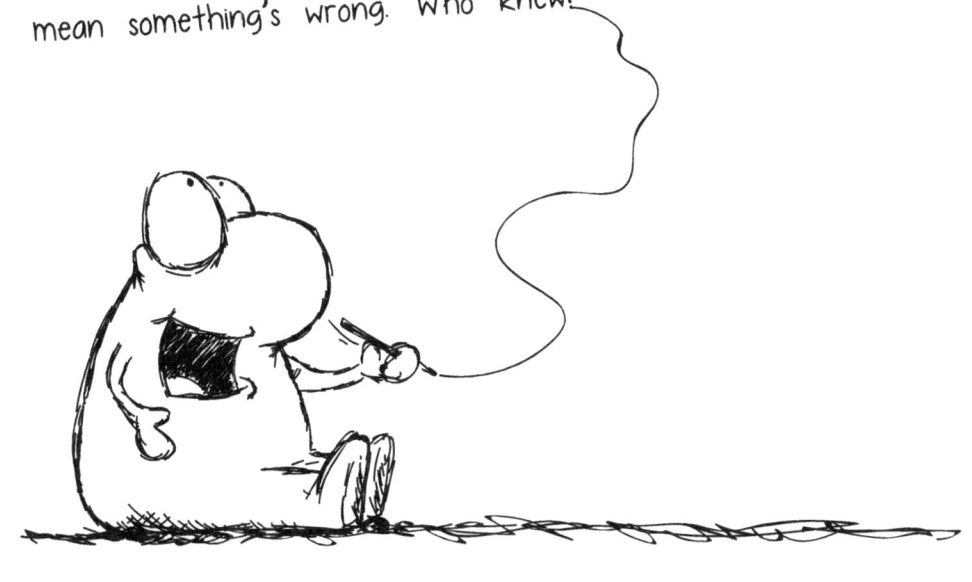

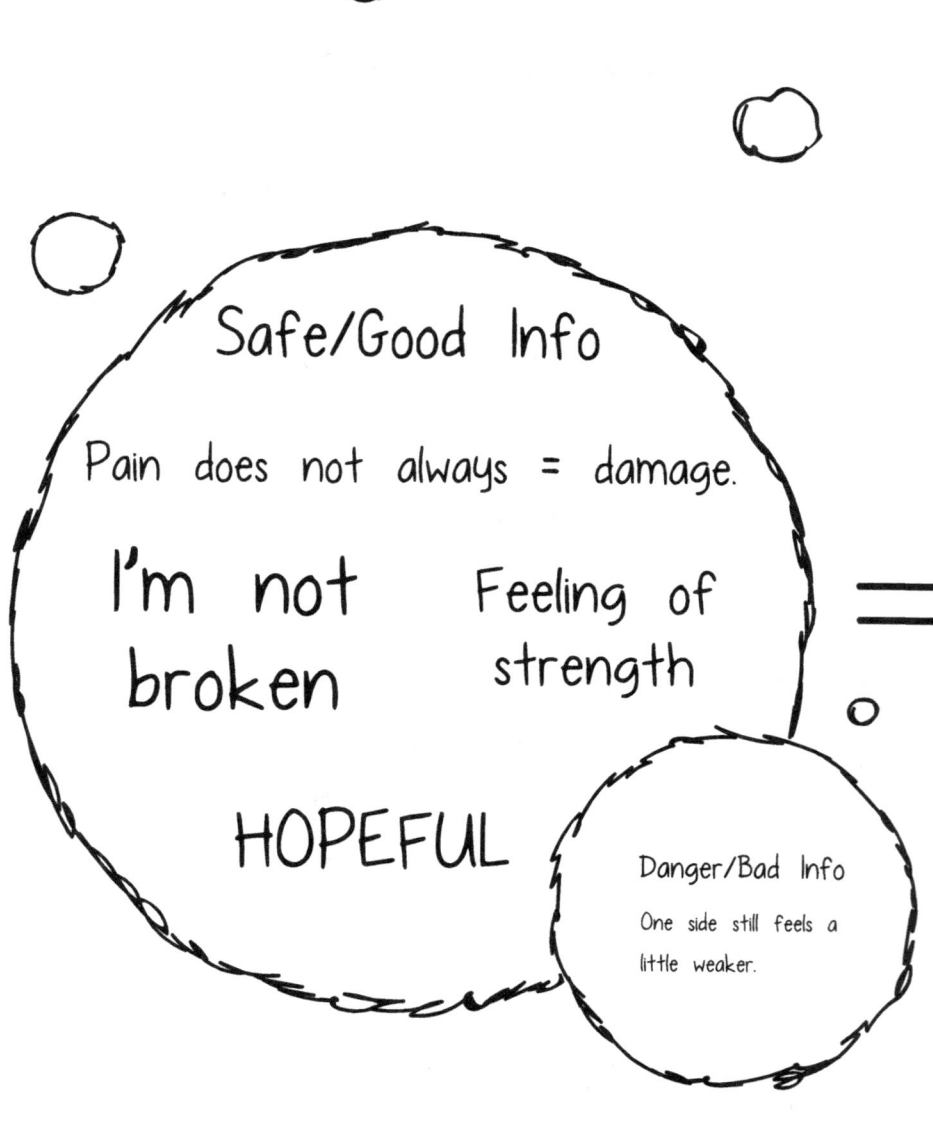

Safe/Good Info

Pain does not always = damage.

I'm not broken

Feeling of strength

HOPEFUL

Danger/Bad Info

One side still feels a little weaker.

Perception

→ "I'm okay, I don't need to protect. I'm excited to see what I can do."

If you have access to a physiotherapist or doctor...

have him or her perform a 1-time assessment to see if there is anything structurally wrong that needs fixing (e.g. broken bone, dislocated hip). If there is, they will treat this. If there isn't, have them confirm whether you have chronic back pain that is ready for the training in this series of books. When you are approved, you are ready to start.

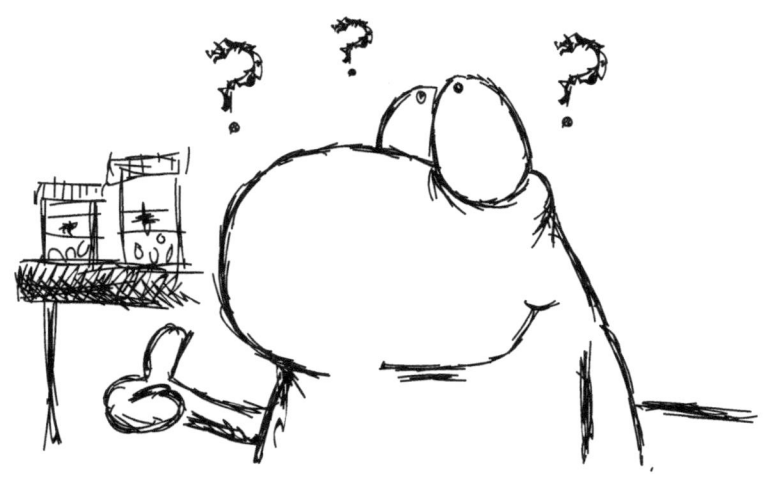

Note. If you have just broken a bone or dislocated a hip, this 4-week program is not for you right now. You need to work with your doctor and/or physio to heal.

However, if your pain continues past the time where your doctor or physio says you should be healed...

and if your doctor or physio has approved you for physical rehab exercises, then this program is right for you.

Important

We will likely believe that bad posture, tight, or weak muscles are the cause of our chronic back pain... because of how our body feels and looks. This has to be one of the reasons for our pain, right?

New research supports that continued pain/a faulty alarm system is the reason for this bad posture, tight, and weak muscles as a protective mechanism... stopping us from doing movements perceived as harmful or wanting to hold the body in a protective posture. Our body may not even have bad posture, weak, or tight muscles, but it may feel like it does because we have put so much attention on one part of the body that our brain makes everything felt from this area a bigger deal...

To recover we need to calm the alarm bells that say we are in danger of an injury. We need to calm those alarm bells so we can once again be free to move in whatever way we choose without thinking about it and so that we no longer have to hold our body in a protective posture.

Note. See the book "Explain Pain" for study references. This book will be the easiest place to understand this research as most journals that have the complete article require a subscription and may be difficult to interpret for those that do not have a research background.

Calming the Alarm Bells Exercises:

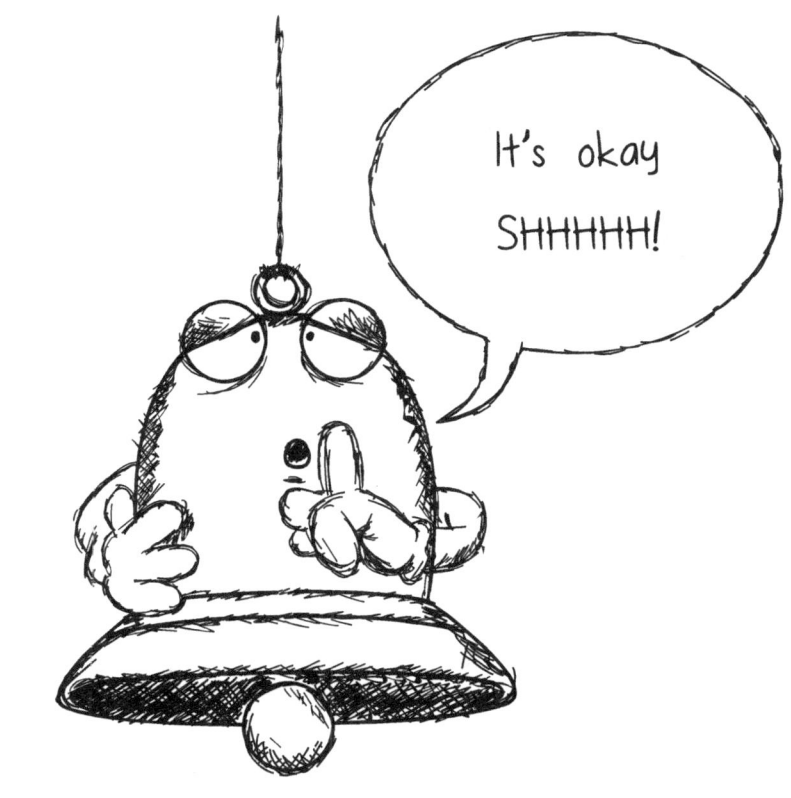

It's okay
SHHHHH!

Exercise 1

Confirming what we know about pain

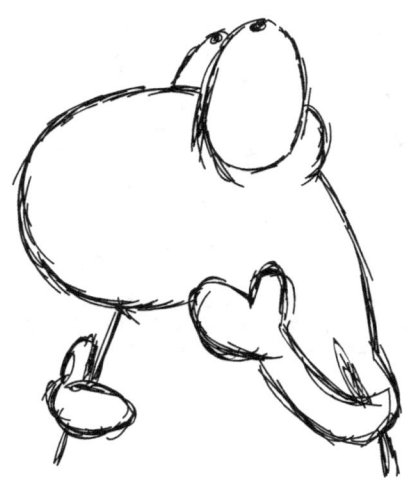

THIS WEEK

Read through each day:

I know now...

- my old belief was: Pain = damage, injury, "something's wrong" (And this may still be present... and that's o.k.)

- my old belief was: Damage always = pain

- my new understanding is: Pain does not always = damage, injury, "something's wrong" and Damage does not always = pain, especially with chronic pain

- I do not have an injury that needs fixing, if a recent diagnosis of something like a broken bone or dislocated hip wasn't found

- with chronic pain I can have "damage" or degeneration and the body can be very capable and without constant pain

Continued...

I know now...

- when I feel the old pain pattern, I am not hurting myself

- bad posture, tight, or weak muscles are not the cause of my chronic pain

- when I feel the old pain pattern, its not because I did something the wrong way

- the reason I have good days is not because I have become stronger, more flexible, and now have better alignment

- the structure of my back is not the reason for my pain

- the reason I keep having back pain is because I have a sensitized nervous system

- there is no reason why I cannot make a full recovery from chronic pain and get back to the activities I love

By confirming each day what we know now about pain, we begin to confront untrue beliefs about pain that say, "something's wrong". We begin to challenge their truthfulness.

Note. We may also have conditions like osteoarthritis or disc degeneration that can limit what activities we can and can't do, and contribute to episodes of pain and inflammation.

However, we can have a full recovery from pain, swelling, and limited activity due to faulty protective or "something's wrong" habits, in the body and mind.

Even with conditions such as osteoarthritis, disc degeneration, and herniated discs, where we have been in pain for a while, sensitivity is at play. As long as there is pain, we know that our danger alarm system is working. We are interpreting that we need to protect, that there is some kind of threat.

Which is good news, because there is no reason why we cannot alleviate the pain, swelling, and limitation of activity due to sensitivty. It is important to know that even with conditions like osteoarthitis, disc degeneration, and herniated discs; it is possible (and common) that all of the pain is due to sensitivity and not the condition itself. So whether some, or all of your chronic pain is due to sensitivity, this 4-week mind/body training will target the pain from sensitivty to help you find ease and comfort again.

Exercise 2

Working from clarity during exercise: knowing when you're in danger of an injury vs. not

THIS WEEK

Every time pain or worry (that something bad is going to happen) comes up, stop and ask:

1. Am I in danger of getting an actual injury right now?

(like a broken bone or dislocated hip)

Yes - stop activity

See a doctor. Let yourself know that to the best of your ability you will take yourself out of harm's way. You can trust yourself to do this.

No - proceed to the next question, but first go through the following...

If there is no feeling like a bone is going to break or a hip is going to dislocate right now, I know now that it's not true that I am in danger of an injury. This is just an old pain pattern playing. I've felt this before. And it's not true anymore.

$\rightarrow$

Note 1. Thinking that something bad is going to happen now, or later on, is not the same as being in danger of an actual injury. This is a worry cycle.

Note 2. Flare-ups (same back pain repeating itself or can't move patterns cycling every couple of months or yearly, and no injury was found on the recent physio assessment) are not actual injuries. This is the sensitivity cycle where we have passed that threshold where we think we are safe and have gone into high alert again. We think we are in danger and we need to protect. This feeling of something is wrong can be subconscious.

2. Am I too worried to continue this activity?

Yes - stop activity

Let yourself know that you will not put yourself in a situation where there is too much worry. (For example: worry about the tension you are experiencing, the worry that happens when you feel weak, or the worry that happens when you think you did something the wrong way... all of which makes you think you are going to hurt yourself). You will stop the activity and extend support, kindness, and compassion to that person who is struggling with worry right now. You will try again tomorrow when the perceived danger is not as high.

No - proceed with activity

This is where there may be a bit of worry still around, but you know theoretically or actually you are not in danger of an injury. Staying in the activity will not be overwhelming with worry.

Each time chronic pain or worry comes up, repeat these questions...

1. Am I in danger of getting an actual injury right now?

2. Am I too worried to continue this activity?

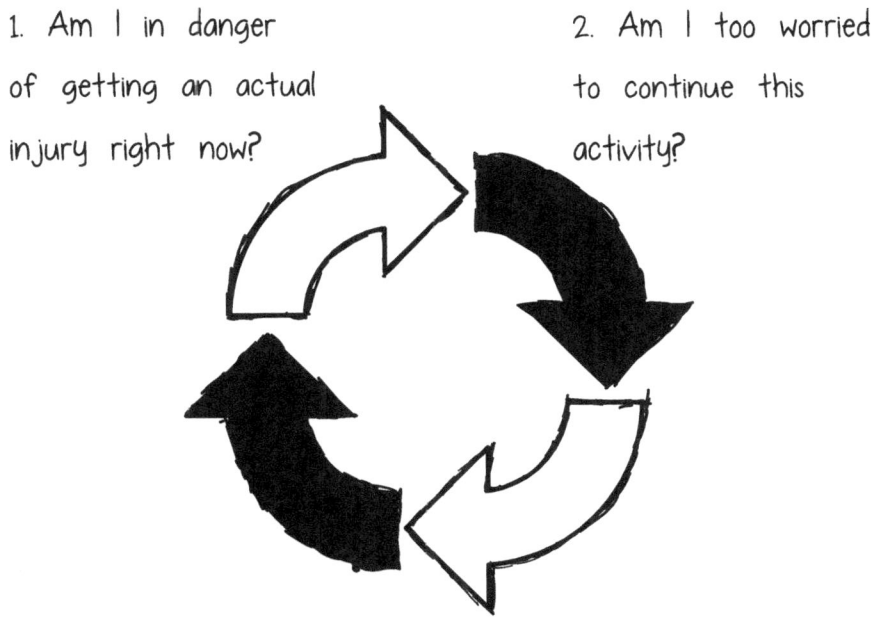

and answer them to know what to do.

This is how we will begin to re-gain trust in our body and ultimately ourselves.

Because we know, that to the best of our ability, we will not put ourselves in a situation that will cause actual harm or will be too overwhelming with worry.

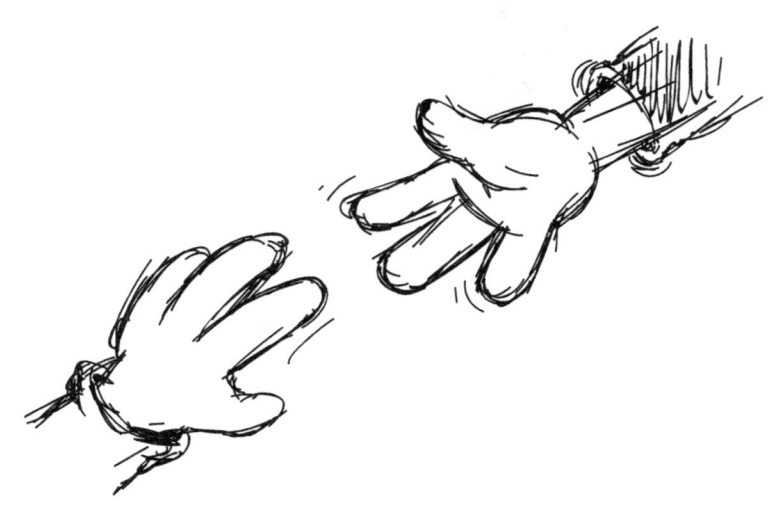

Note. I hope from this chapter we can begin to see that this is not simply positive thinking. We are not here to say there is no danger every time pain or worry comes up. This is about working from what is actually happening. We will have to slow down each time worry or pain comes up to see if it's true that we are in danger of an injury. This is about drawing from knowledge of pain and our direct experience to inform our decision-making, actions... our entire being.

I recommend reading the book "Explain Pain" over the next few weeks to better understand pain.

by David Butler and Lorimer Moseley. 2nd ed. Adelaide: NOI Group Publications; 2013.

Before reading on...

give yourself a moment to think
on this chapter.

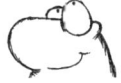

CHAPTER 2

Re-discovering our body's power, capability, and skillfulness

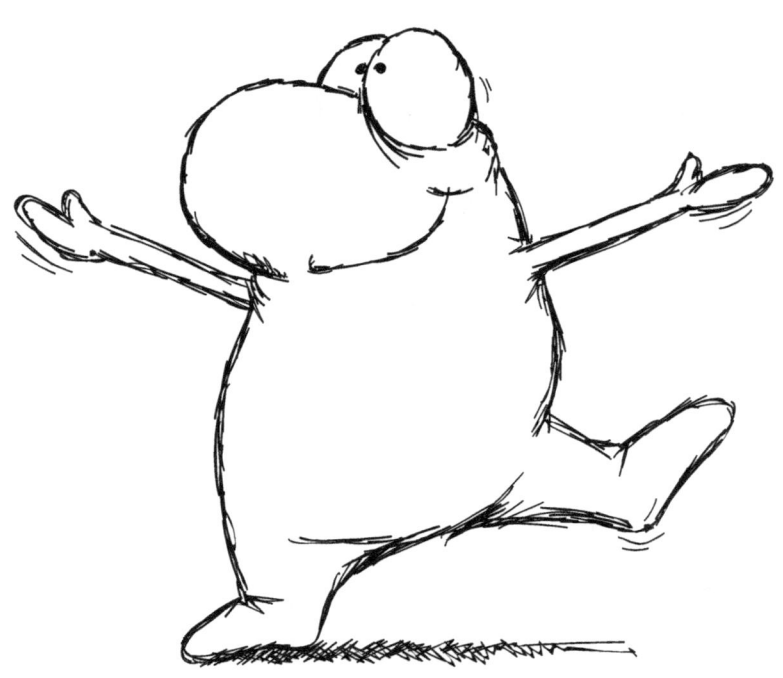

The following is the exercise for Week 1, in a series of a 4-week program. Each week a new exercise will be introduced.

The 4 exercises were selected to first help dissolve any protective patterns for our back (like tucking under or guarding) by finding a way of moving that brings a sense of power, capability, and skillfulness. All of which will tell our brain, and entire being, that we are o.k. We don't need to protect.

Once we have reduced or dissolved the feeling of vulnerability, hesitation to move, or need to protect; the later weeks will focus on strengthening so we can take on more difficult challenges.

Remember, the reason for strengthening is not to get us out of pain (e.g. we are not in pain because we are weak). No matter whether we have had pain or not, we strengthen our bodies to get us ready to do a new activity or one that hasn't been done in a while... so we are ready to take on the challenge. For now, let's focus on dissolving our protective patterns with the help of Exercise 1.

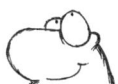

Exercise 1: Side Leg Lifts

Let's do a couple of leg lifts on
each side so we can see how
they feel.

Side Leg Lifts

End
Position

Start
Position

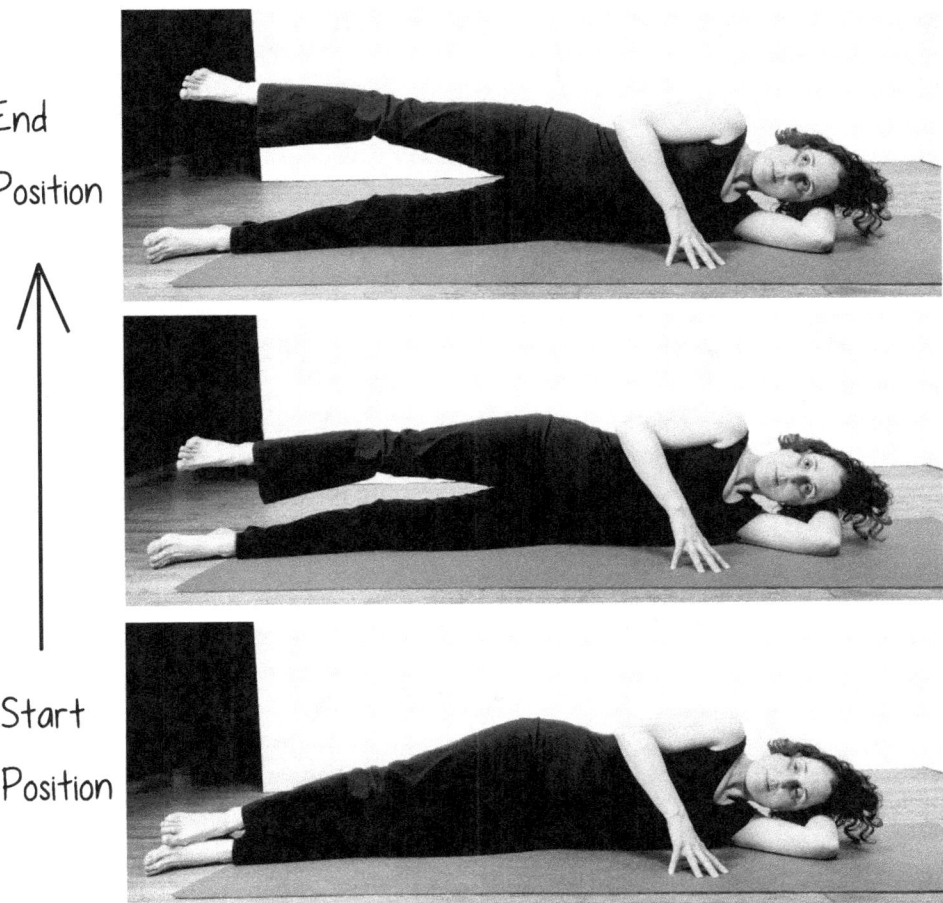

Lift and lower the leg

If there is any discomfort, only lift the
top leg a little for now.

So did we do them right?

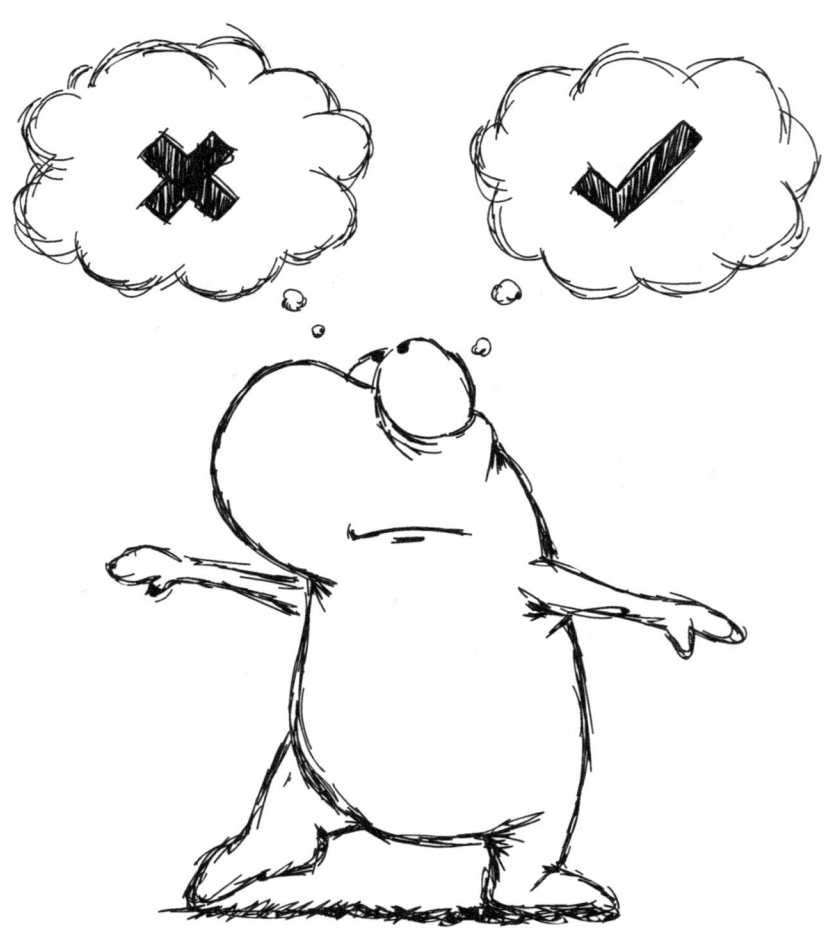

Let's find out...

What likely happened

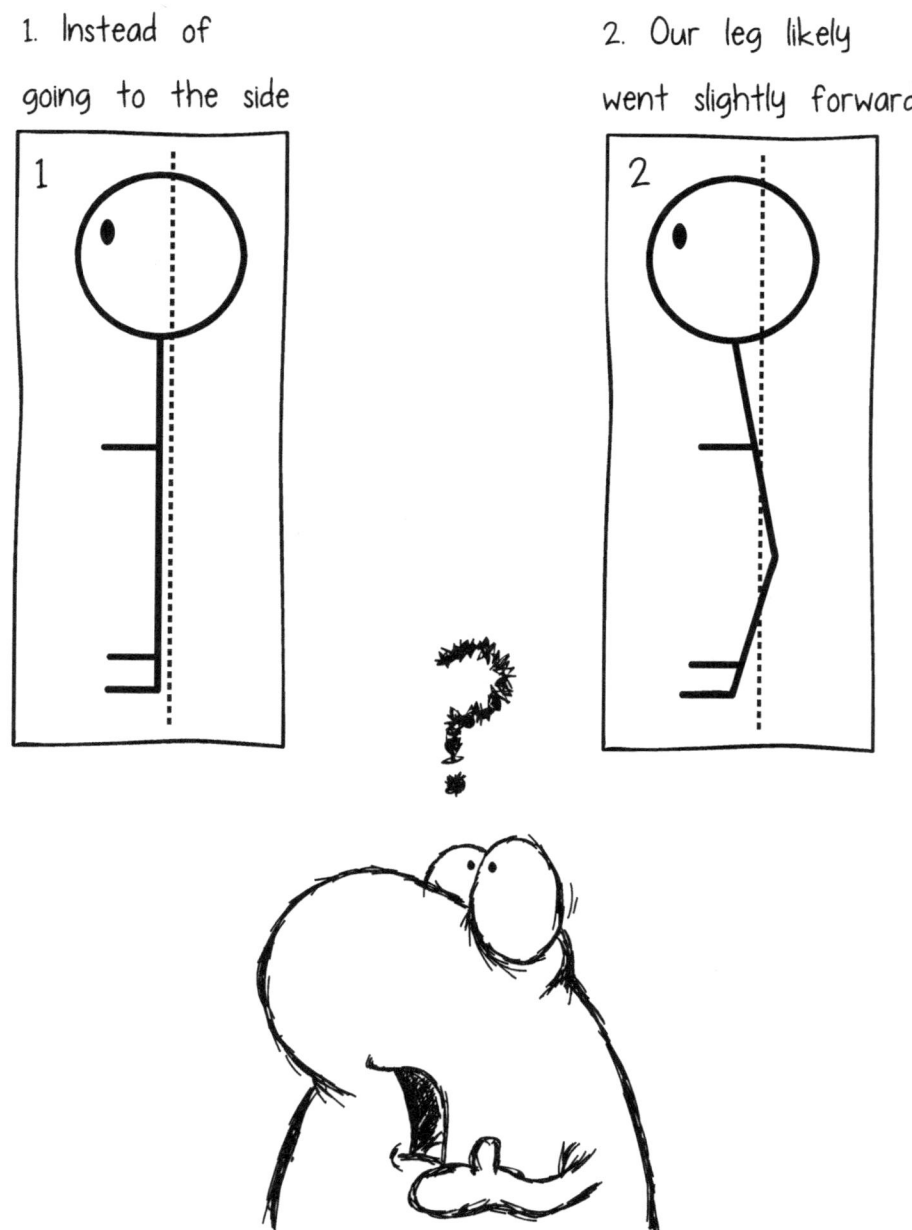

1. Instead of going to the side

2. Our leg likely went slightly forward

Let's try another leg lift to see
if our leg went forward.

Don't correct anything! We need
to see how we move first. See
the next page for what to look
for...

While lying on our right side,
let's look down.

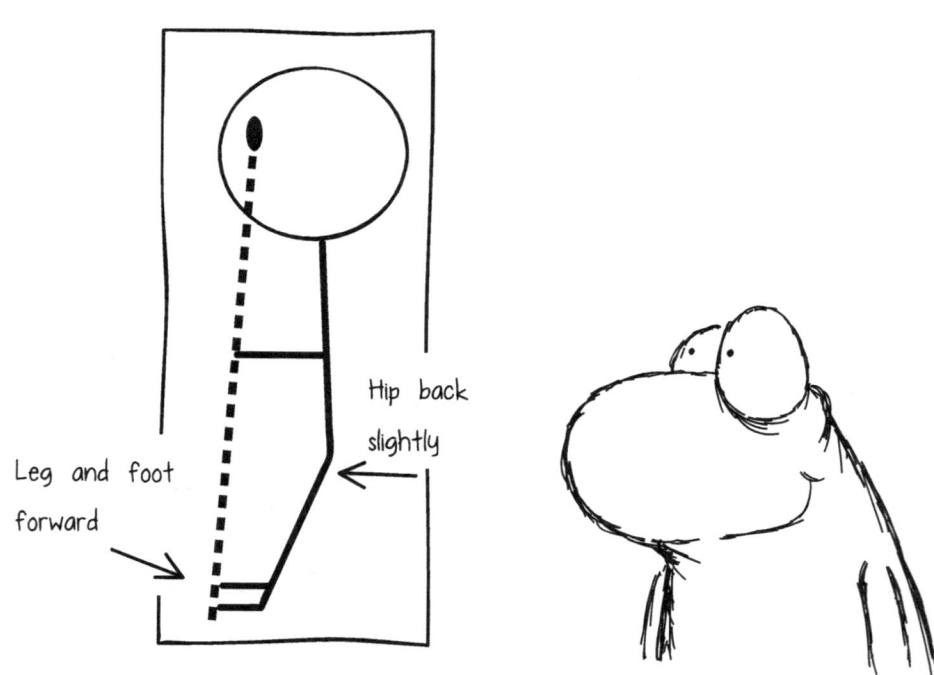

Hip back
slightly

Leg and foot
forward

Here's what to look for:
If we can see our toes, our leg
is slightly forward already. This will
continue in the leg lift. This is
called "hip flexion."

Why does it matter if our leg goes forward?

When our leg goes forward, this means we are really good at using the front of our body, our "flexors." How did we become good at this?...

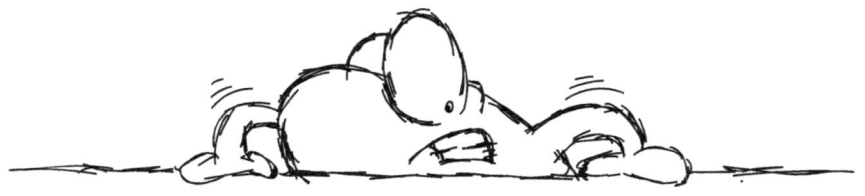

When we are hunched over a lot (holding the weight of our body) or are tucking the pelvis under to flatten and protect our back, the front of the body is mainly working in a particular way. We then usually take this way of moving and holding into all activities.... because we are really good at it and/or it's a posture we feel safe in!

Front of body working in certain ways.

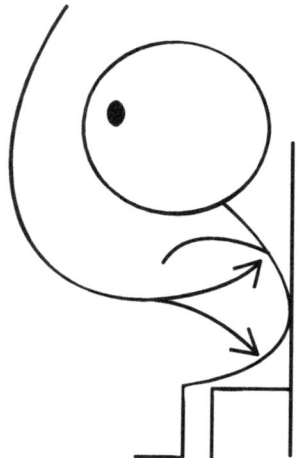 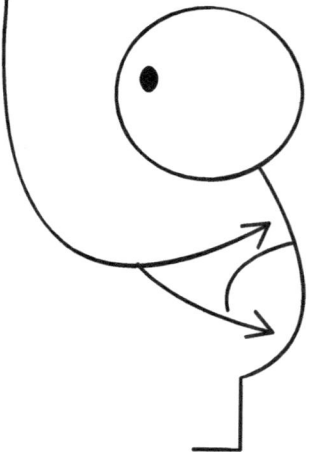

The back of our body is not participating very much at what it does best... extension.

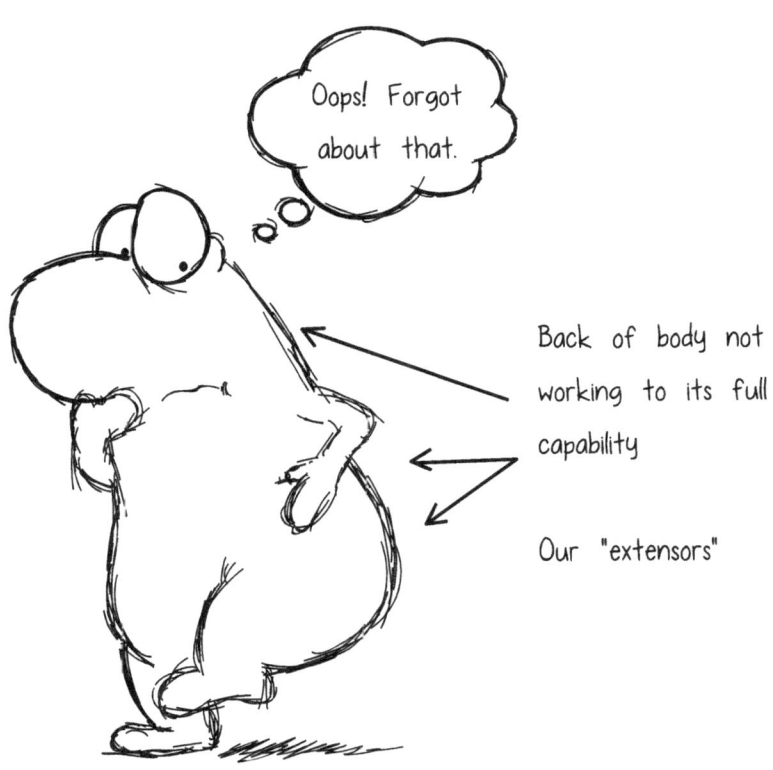

Back of body not working to its full capability

Our "extensors"

This week we are going to re-learn how to use the back of our body again to its full potential.

Accessing the full potential of the muscles on the back of our body, as well as continuing to use the front, will bring a feeling of strength, lightness, comfort, and power.

All of which will tell our brain, and entire being, that we are o.k.

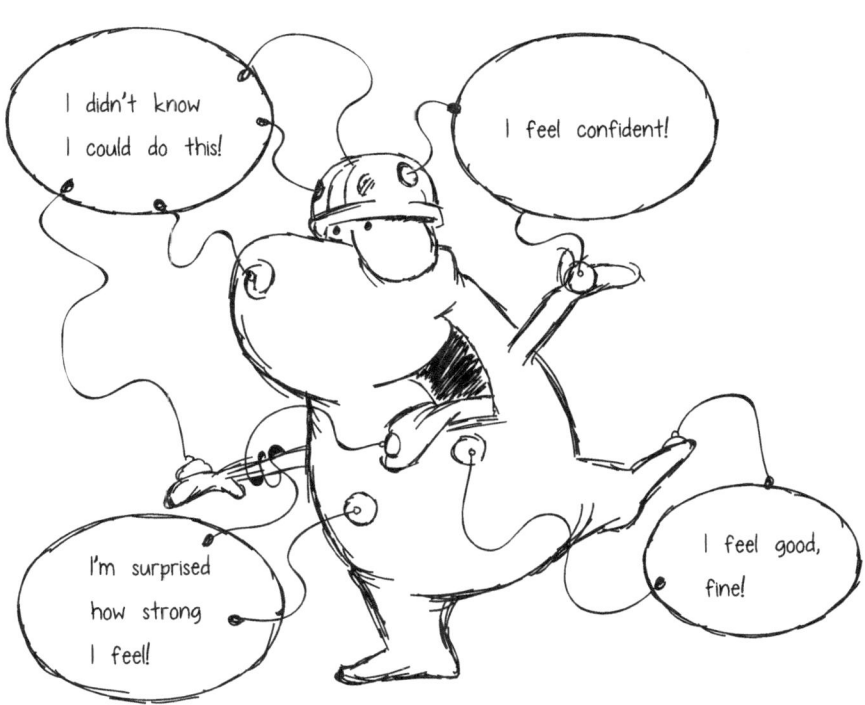

Since we already have the qualities of strength, lightness, power, and comfort; (they have just been dimmed from our attention on the constant pain, exhaustion, and frustration) we can access these qualities we love on our first day. We just need to re-learn how to find them and take time to feel them.

* Important *

Doing the leg lifts "wrong" will not hurt us.

My clients often ask if they are doing their exercises "right." So I will work with this language because it seems easier to relate to by most people. Doing the leg lifts "right" will mean we have the technique for re-developing the full potential of our body (we are allowing all ways of moving and they are supported, strong, yet fluid; we are not protecting).

To be clear, I am not linking our chronic back pain with doing the leg lifts the wrong way or bad posture... as the reason for our pain.

How to use the back of our body

→ Have a look
while I demonstrate.
I will do "Hip Extension."

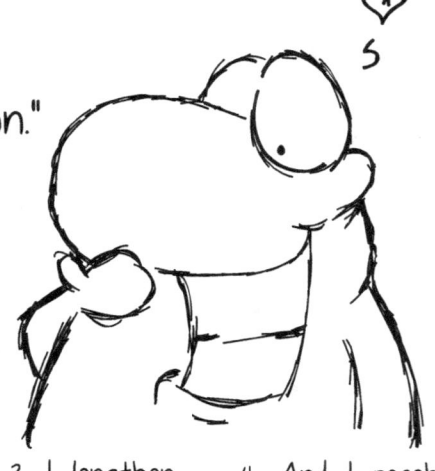

1. I lie on
my side

2. My hip goes
forward

3. I lengthen
my leg out
to my foot

4. And I reach
my lower thigh
and leg back

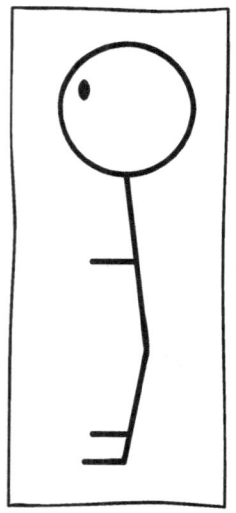

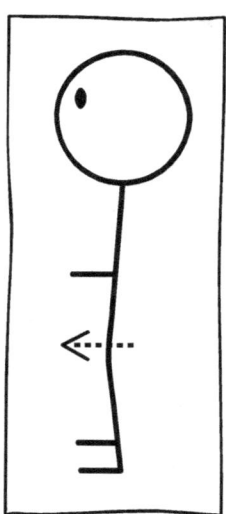

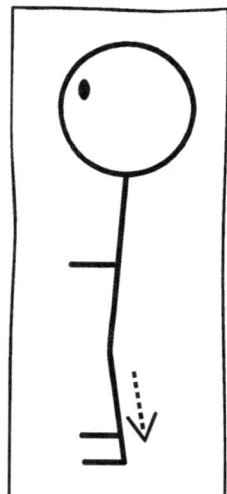

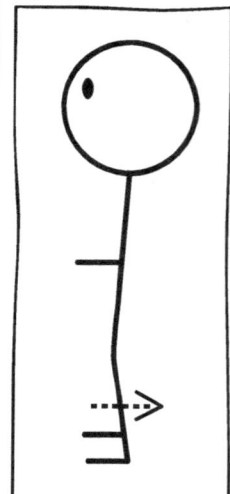

The muscles working now are on the back of the body...

Hip Extension

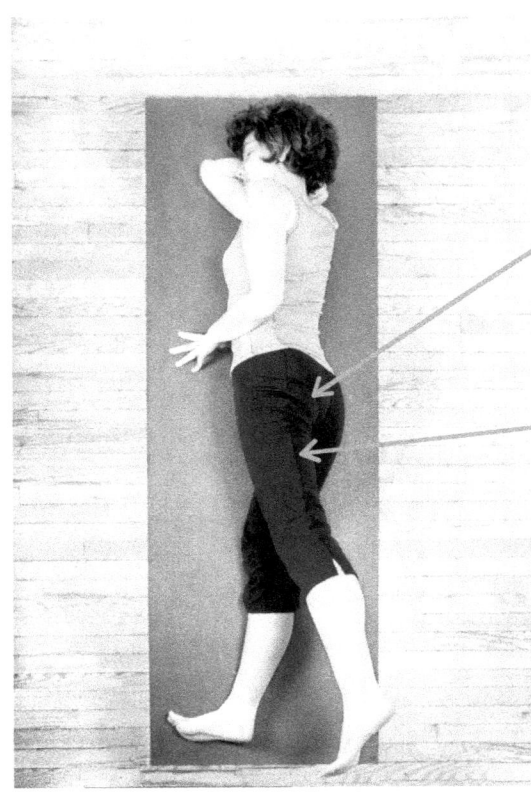

Back of the buttocks, or "glutes" firm

Back of the thigh or "hamstrings" firm

Note. The bottom leg/foot is reaching into the ground to help us balance and lift the top leg up away from the bottom leg. It can be surprising how hard the bottom leg is working.

Why haven't we been using these muscles?

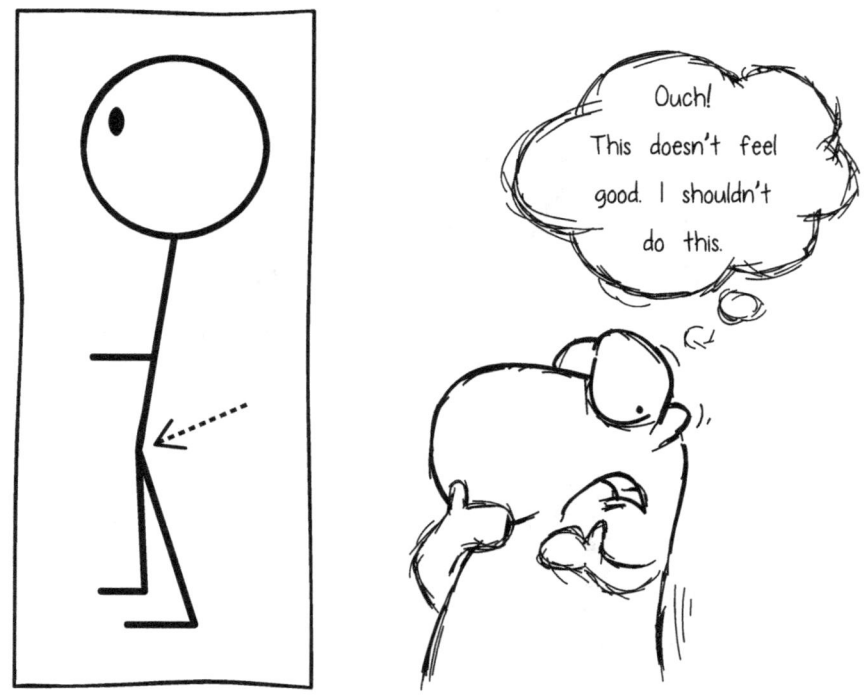

When we do our hip extension, our low back curve becomes more arched. As a result, our low back will likely feel vulnerable. So we stay away from this type of movement.

Note. Remember our back is not actually vulnerable to injury here, in hip extension. It can just feel like it. This is where we can feel unsafe and the pain/tension that continually comes with this posture makes it feel true that we are hurting ourselves. It becomes like a self-fulfilling prophecy, "see I told you I would get that pain if I did that. I can't do that movement." Remember, pain does not always equal injury/something's wrong.

What we need to re-learn, is how to support our low back while we do this hip extension so we can feel lightness, strength, power, and comfort with this movement again.

Here's how...

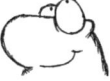

How to support our low back

→ Keep watching while I demonstrate.

"Top-of-the-tailbone work"

1. While I am doing hip extension...

2. I move the top of my tailbone down and forward

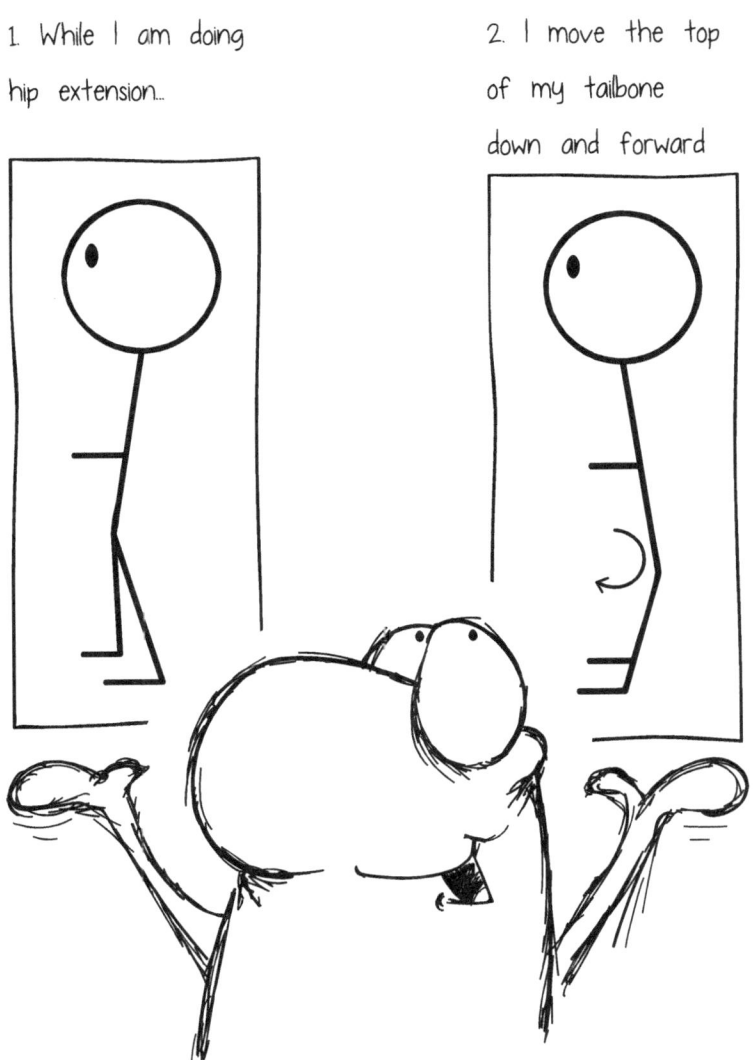

Note. The tailbone is the lowest part of our spine, which can be found between the lower portion of the buttocks muscles.

The result

When we move the top of the tailbone down and firm it forward, our low back gets a little longer (or you could say a little flatter).

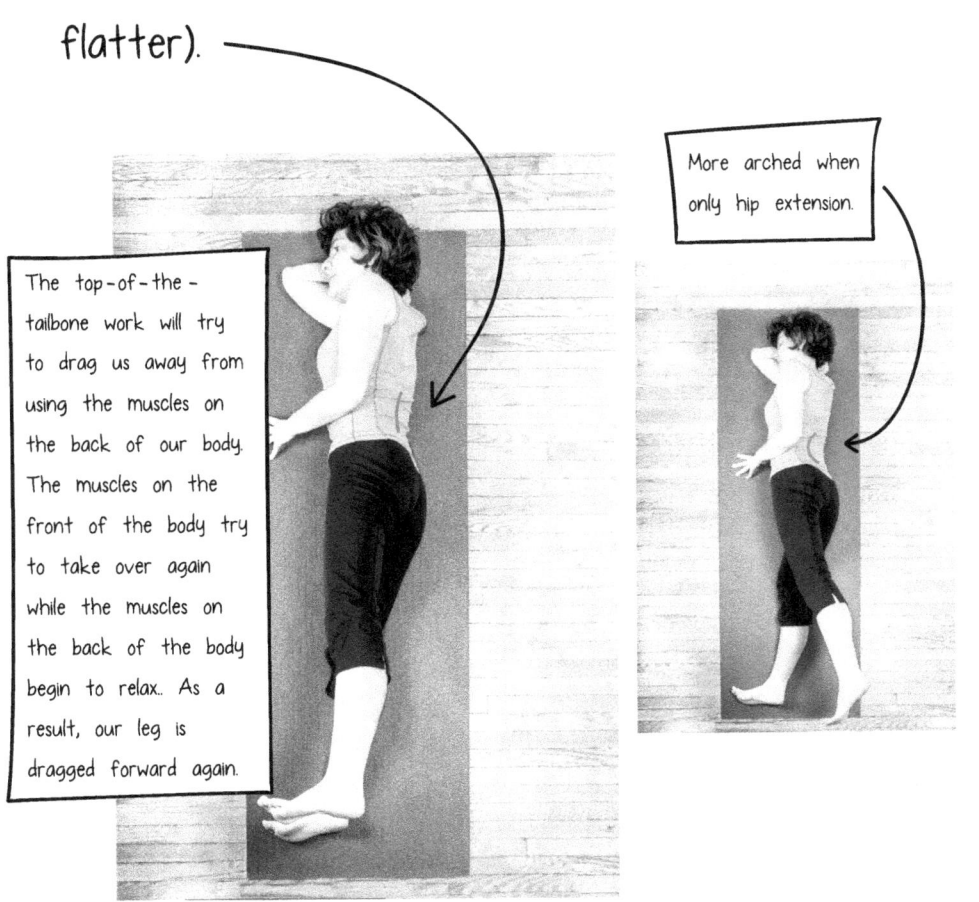

More arched when only hip extension.

The top-of-the-tailbone work will try to drag us away from using the muscles on the back of our body. The muscles on the front of the body try to take over again while the muscles on the back of the body begin to relax. As a result, our leg is dragged forward again.

This is because it is the opposite action of hip extension.

So we must learn how to keep both at the same time!

1. Hip extension

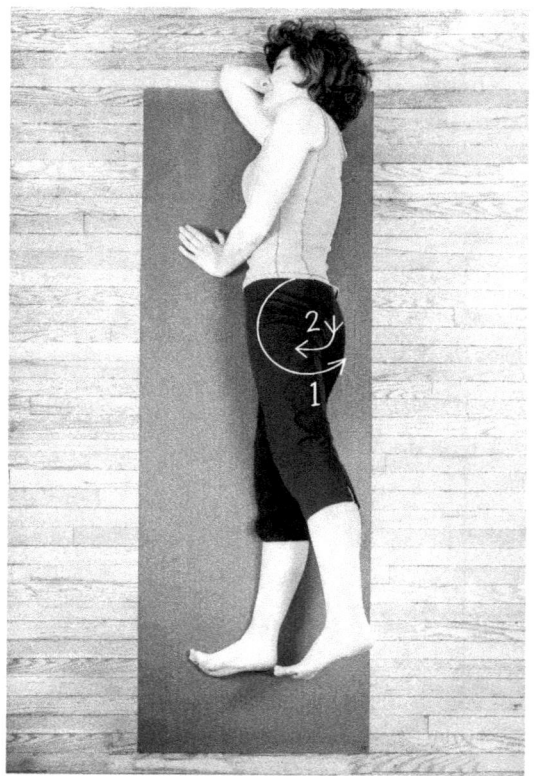

2. While we maintain the top-of-the-tailbone work

This way, the back of the body will have to work even harder to keep hip extension... which is good. And our backs will feel no discomfort as we keep them supported with the top-of-the-tailbone work.

Now let's have you try...

Start by lying on your right side.

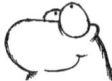

Try hip extensions 2 to 3 times

Follow the 4 steps below
to complete hip extension...

1. Lie on your side

2. Move your front hip point forward

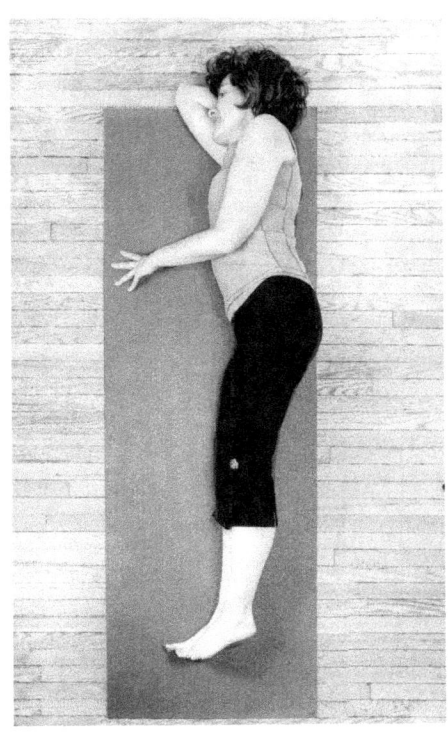

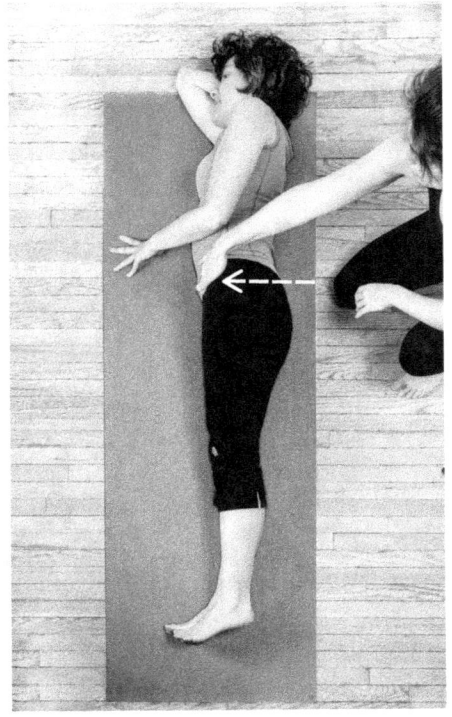

Note. If lying on the floor feels uncomfortable, see pg 160 for different ways to set-up the exercise for comfort.

3. Lengthen your leg out to your foot

4. Reach your lower thigh and leg back

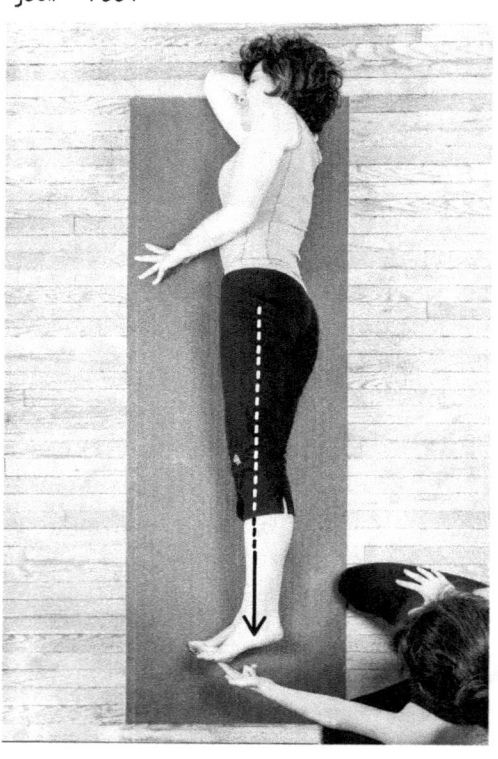

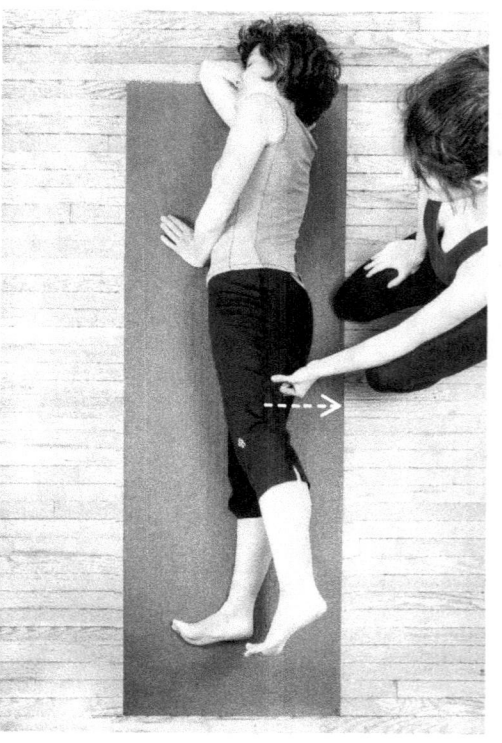

If your back hurts a little with this movement, don't reach your leg as far back. If your back still hurts a little, don't lift the top leg up off the bottom leg. This will make hip extension an even smaller movement and challenge.

Rest back down for a couple of breaths.

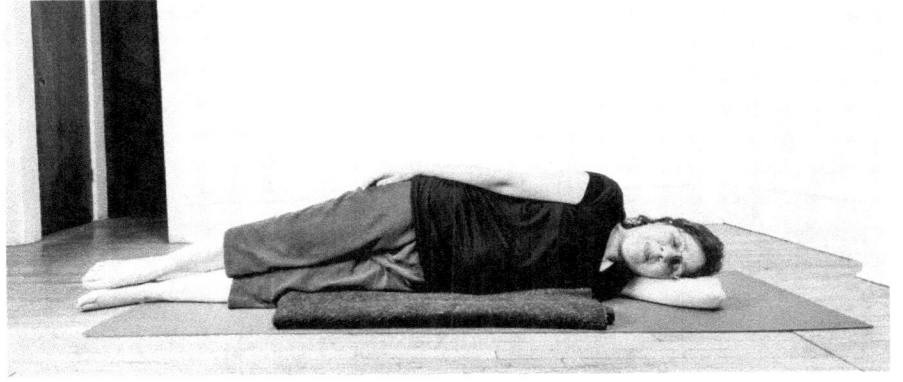

If you're comfortable to do so, allow your eyes to close. Feel your natural in-breath at your nose (or mouth if this feel more comfortable), and your natural out-breath. Just rest and breathe...

If any pain, stiffness, feeling weak, or worry has come up from this movement, read pages 153 - 157 in the Summary chapter now. And only proceed with the exercise today if the worry, pain, or bad sensations have eased a little.

Did you do it right?

If you felt:

✓ Low back curve arched a bit more

✓ Back of buttocks muscles firm

✓ and the muscles on the back of your thigh firm

Yes... you got it.

IF you're not sure those things happened, let me help you figure this out.

Note 1. You are not trying to firm your buttocks or increase your low back curve, they just happen as a result of doing hip extension. 2. You will also feel the muscle on the side of your hip (a glute muscle) working because this is what lifts the leg up away from the floor and controls the leg when it is lowered down. This is separate from doing hip extension.

You will first need to do it "wrong" so you can feel the difference.

Do hip flexion...

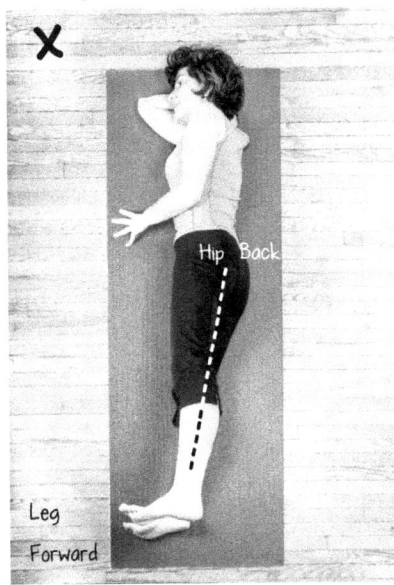

Then do hip extension...

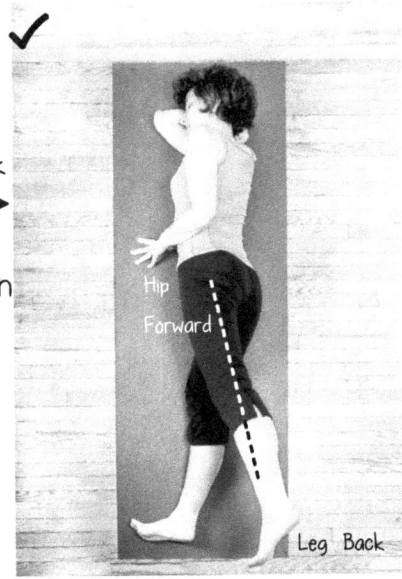

Back →
← Forth

Can you feel:
-low back curve flatter
-muscles on front of hip and thigh firming (muscles on back of buttocks slightly stretching or relaxing)

Can you feel:
-low back curve a little more arched
-muscles on back of the buttocks and thigh firming (muscles on front of hip and thigh slightly stetching or relaxing)

Remember, you won't hurt yourself if you do it "wrong"... these are very gentle exercises.

Swing gently from hip flexion to extension (holding each for a few seconds) 2 to 3 times so you can feel the difference.

Once you can feel the difference, you will know when you are in hip extension and when you are not.

Rest for a couple of breaths again.

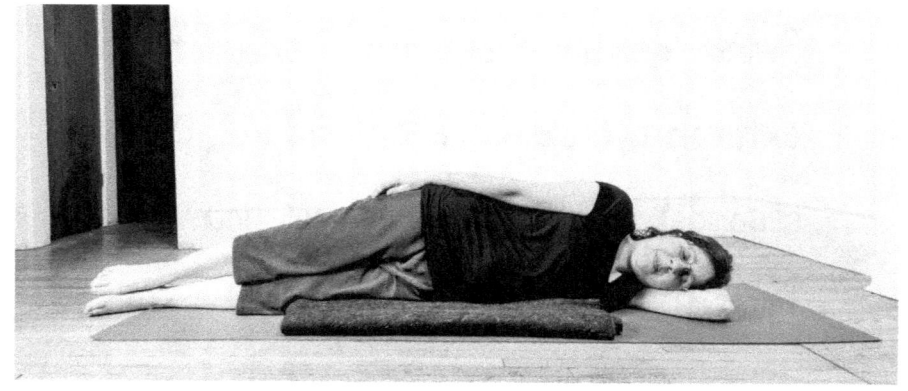

If you're comfortable to do so, allow your eyes to close. Feel your natural in-breath at your nose (or mouth if this feel more comfortable), and your natural out-breath. Just rest and breathe...

If any pain, stiffness, feeling weak, or worry has come up from this movement, read pages 153 - 157 in the Summary chapter now. And only proceed with the exercise today if the worry, pain, or bad sensations have eased a little.

What is likely taking you out of hip extension...

When you reach your leg back, you might be dragging your hip back too....

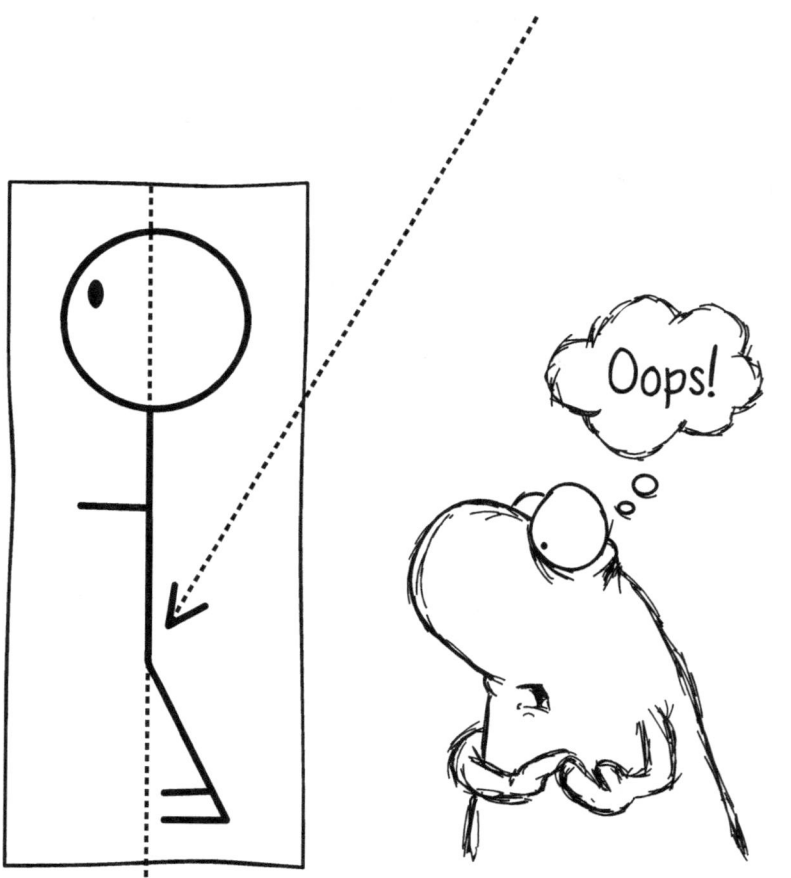

To keep hip extension you must:

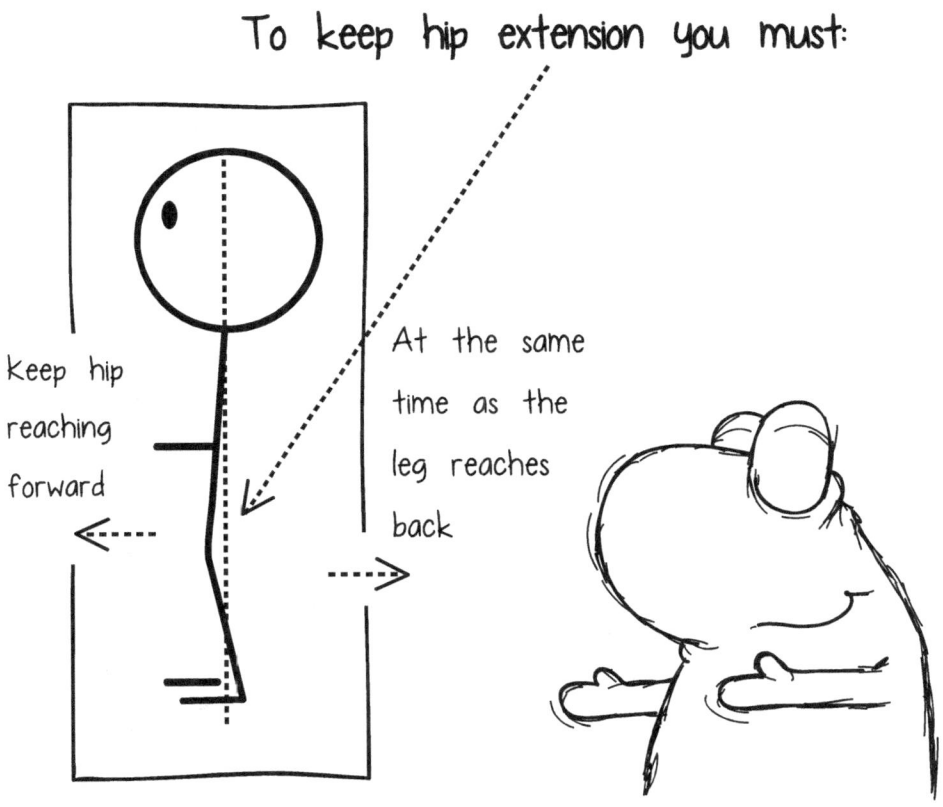

Keep hip reaching forward

At the same time as the leg reaches back

Clients often ask, how much should they reach their hip forward... and how much should they reach their leg back. And I always say... there is no perfect amount. You must go back to what you feel. Does your low back curve arch a bit more, do the muscles on the back of the body start firming? If so, you got it. If your back really feels uncomfortable, then reach your hip a little less forward or your leg a little less back. Do the least amount of these movements that give you the results of hip extension.

Two examples of keeping hip forward at the same time as leg reaches back...

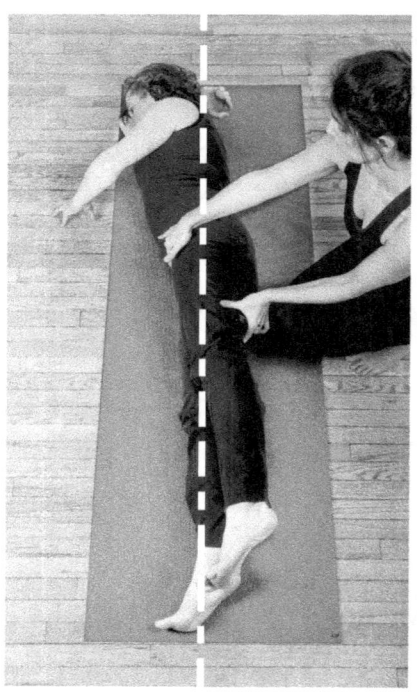 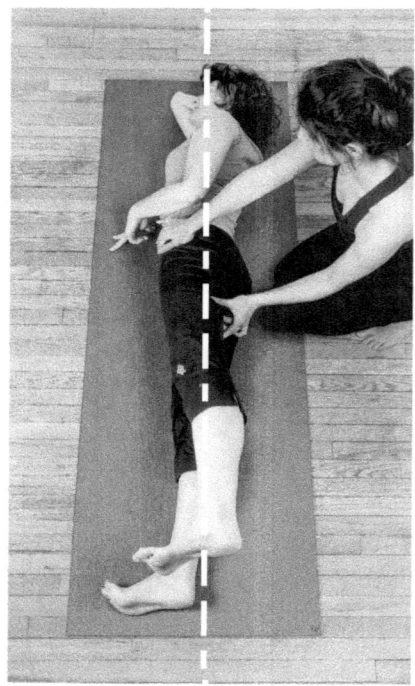

Note. It's o.k. if your upper body goes forward or back... let's just focus on mastering hip extension... maintaining hip forward and leg slightly back.

That's hip extension.

Now let's see how we support our low back....

Stay lying on the right side...

*Before reading on, make sure that you can find hip extension in your body. Give yourself some time to practice.

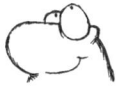

Using the top of our tailbone to support the low back

First... Where is it?

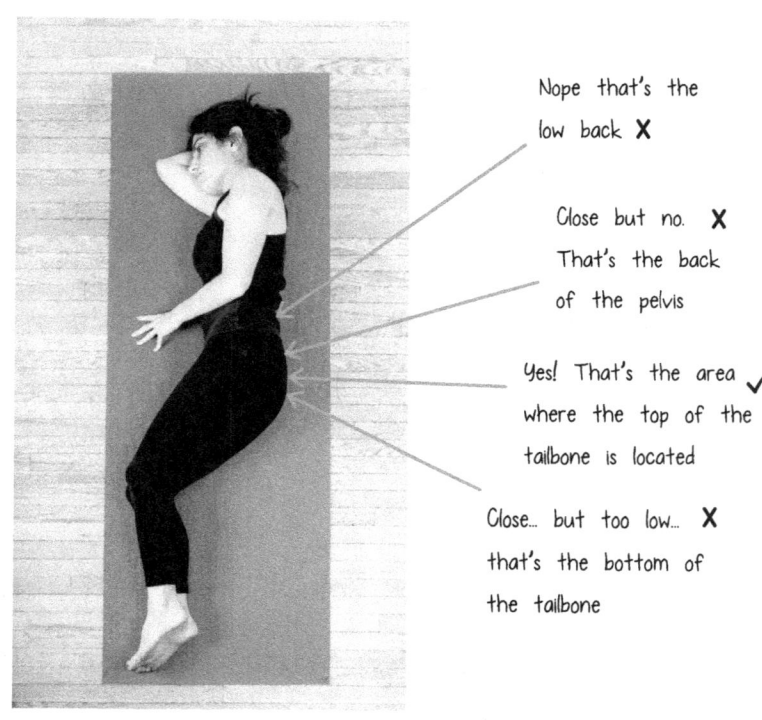

Nope that's the low back **X**

Close but no. **X** That's the back of the pelvis

Yes! That's the area ✓ where the top of the tailbone is located

Close... but too low... **X** that's the bottom of the tailbone

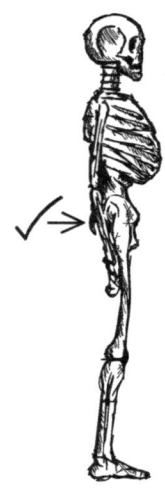

Note. Don't worry about finding the "exact" spot. As long as you are in the area you are good.

Try doing the top-of-the-tailbone work 2 or 3 times

Follow the 3 steps below to complete
the top-of-the-tailbone work...

(keep your legs together, resting down on the floor throughout)

1. Lie on your side

2. Move the top of your tailbone down and firm it forward

3. Relax again

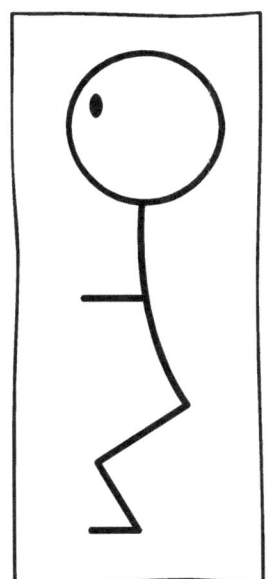 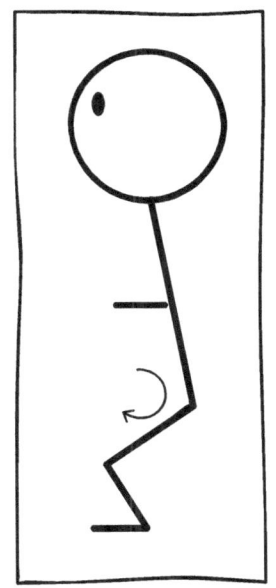 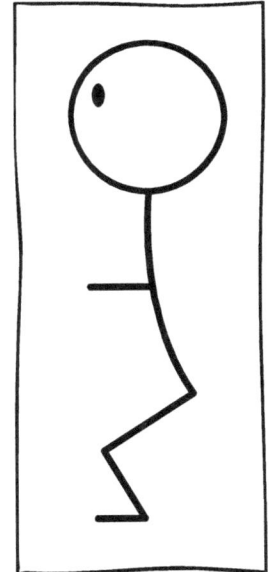

This one can be a bit tougher
to find or feel. Don't worry...
I will help you. Keep reading...

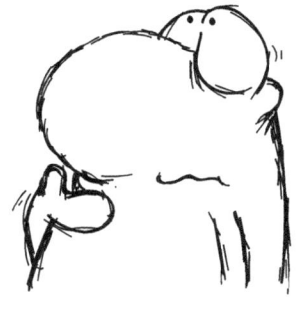

Did you do it right?

If you felt:

✓ Lower abdominals firm
✓ Low back gets a little longer/flatter
✓ and low back feels more supported or
a feeling of lift

Yes... you got it!

IF you're not sure those things happened,
let me help you figure this out.

Note. You are not trying to flatten your back. The low back just slightly lengthens and the abdominals firm as a result of doing top-of-the-tailbone work.

You will first need to do it "wrong" so you can feel the difference.

Release the tip of your tailbone out behind you...

Then move the top of your tailbone down and firm it forward...

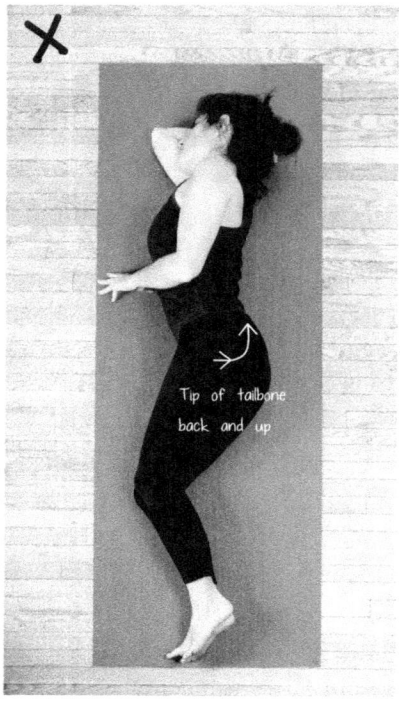

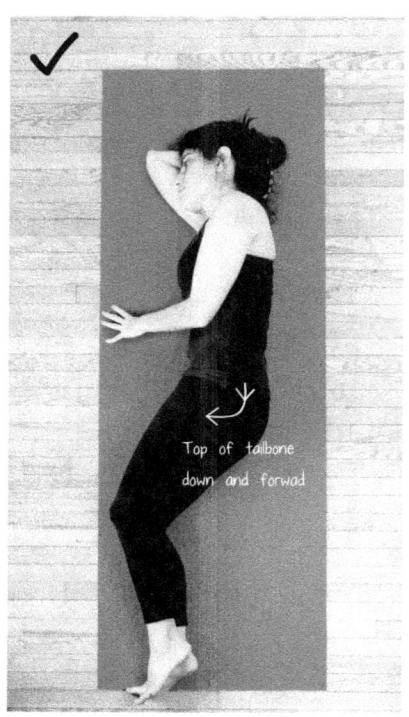

Back
→
←
Forth

Can you feel:
-low back gets more arched
-buttocks sticks out behind you
-lower abs relax and drop to your feet and out behind you

Can you feel:
-low back curve a little longer or you could say flatter
-lower abs become firm

Note. The pictures on the previous page show the extremes of the movement so you can visually see what happens. For our purposes, the top-of-the-tailbone work will be much smaller.

Move gently from one to the other (tip of the tailbone releasing out behind you to working the top of the tailbone down and forward) holding each for a few seconds. Do this 2 to 3 times so you can feel the difference.

Once you can feel the difference you will know when you have the top-of-the-tailbone support for your back and when you don't.

What to watch for:

"Tuck" under

→ Clients often say this when I teach the top-of-the-tailbone work...

If this is what you know, you can start with this idea. The rotation of the pelvis/hips when you "tuck" under is the same direction of rotation that the top-of-the-tailbone work produces. The top-of-the-tailbone work is just a much, much, much smaller action/rotation (which will be needed to allow your body to also do hip extension later on).

Look below to see how small a movement the top-of-the-tailbone work is...

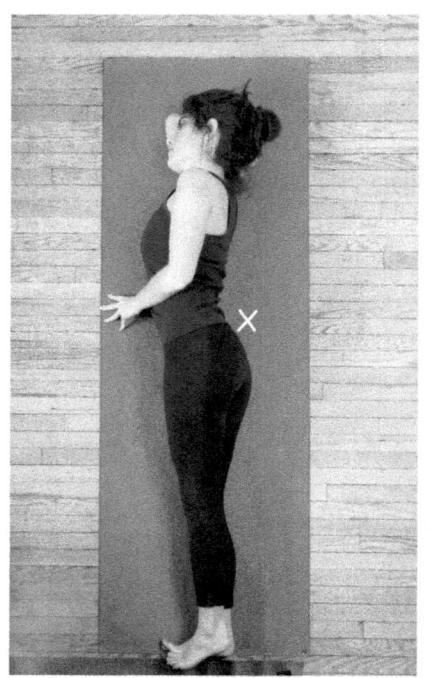
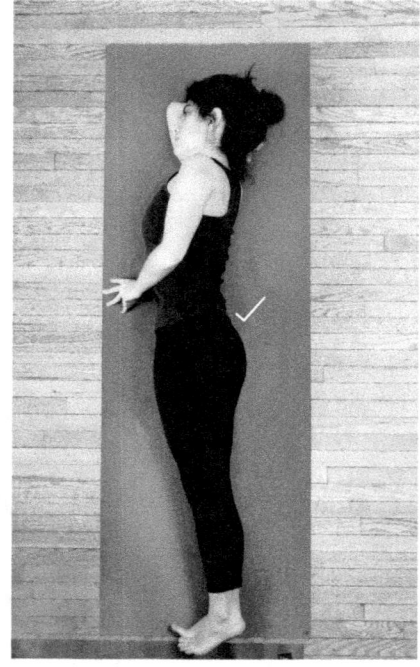

Note. For many people, they won't be able to see the difference between these two photos... and that's o.k.! But, everyone will be able to feel the difference with practice.

That's the top-of-the-tailbone work.

Now let's learn how to put the 2 movements together...

Stay lying on the right side...

*Before reading on, make sure you can find the top-of-the-tailbone work. Give yourself some time to practice.

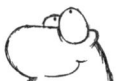

Getting into Position

Try combining the 2 movements,
3 or 4 times.

Why?

Because if you do one action, and
the equal and opposite action at the
same time...

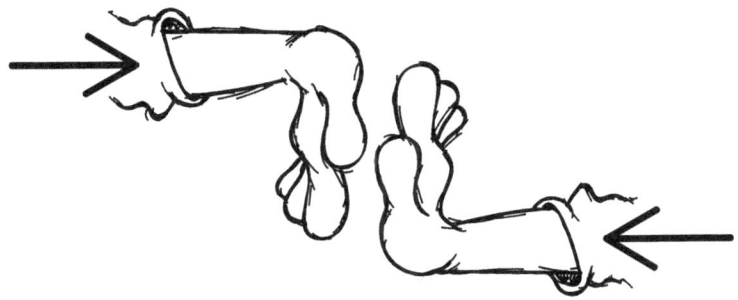

...you will get the feeling of strength, lightness, power, and comfort.

All of which will tell your brain, and entire being, that you are o.k.

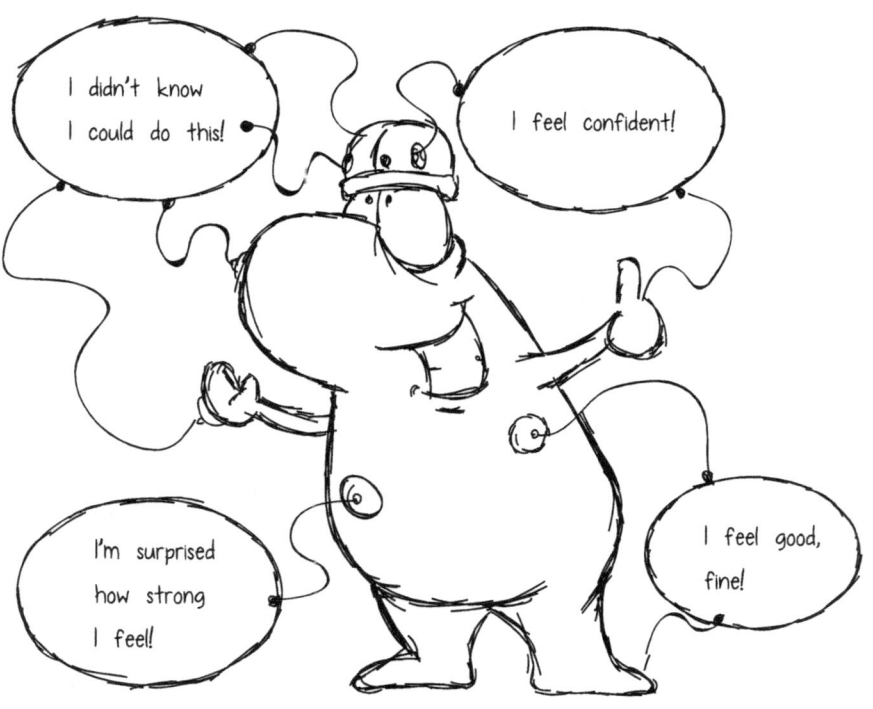

Start by doing...

Hip Extension

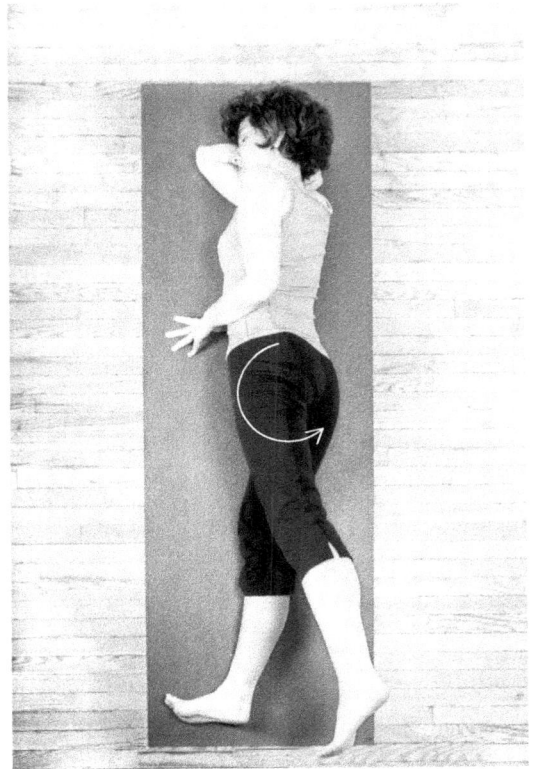

The main movement

Add in...

A little bit of top-of-tailbone work...

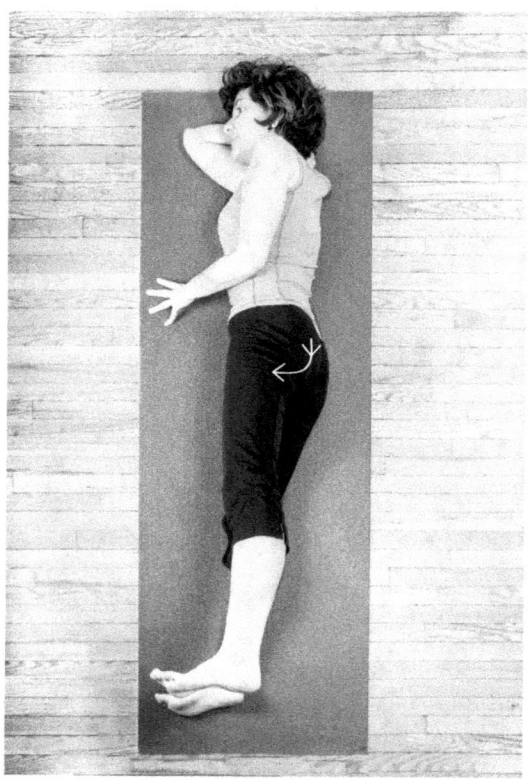

(Opposite movement to hip extension)

Did you feel...

$\longrightarrow$ Often when you add the
top-of-the-tailbone work, it drags
your leg a little forward (and likely
your hip a bit back).

If so, you will need to...

1. Re-strengthen hip extension

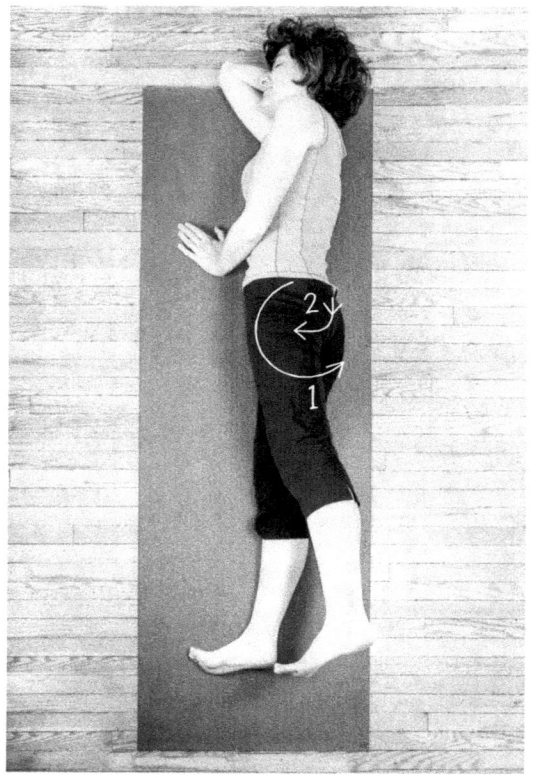

2. While you maintain the top-of-the-tailbone work

Note. The main action is hip extension. Do the littlest amount of top-of-the-tailbone work that will resist it, so your back stays supported.

Rest for a couple of breaths again.

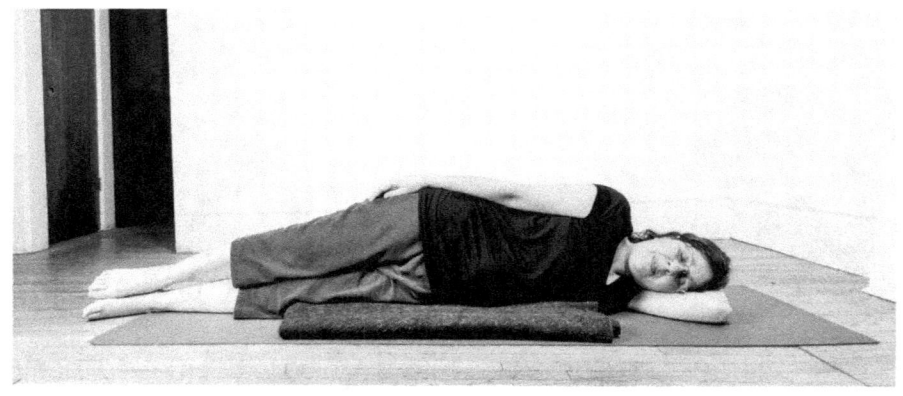

If you're comfortable to do so, allow your eyes to close. Feel your natural in-breath at your nose (or mouth if this feel more comfortable), and your natural out-breath. Just rest and breathe...

If any pain, stiffness, feeling weak, or worry has come up from this movement, read pages 153 - 157 in the Summary chapter now. And only proceed with the exercise today if the worry, pain, or bad sensations have eased a little.

What will likely happen...

You will do one thing, and then lose the other. And vice versa. You will teeter-totter from one to the other!

Back-and-forth Wheeeeeee!

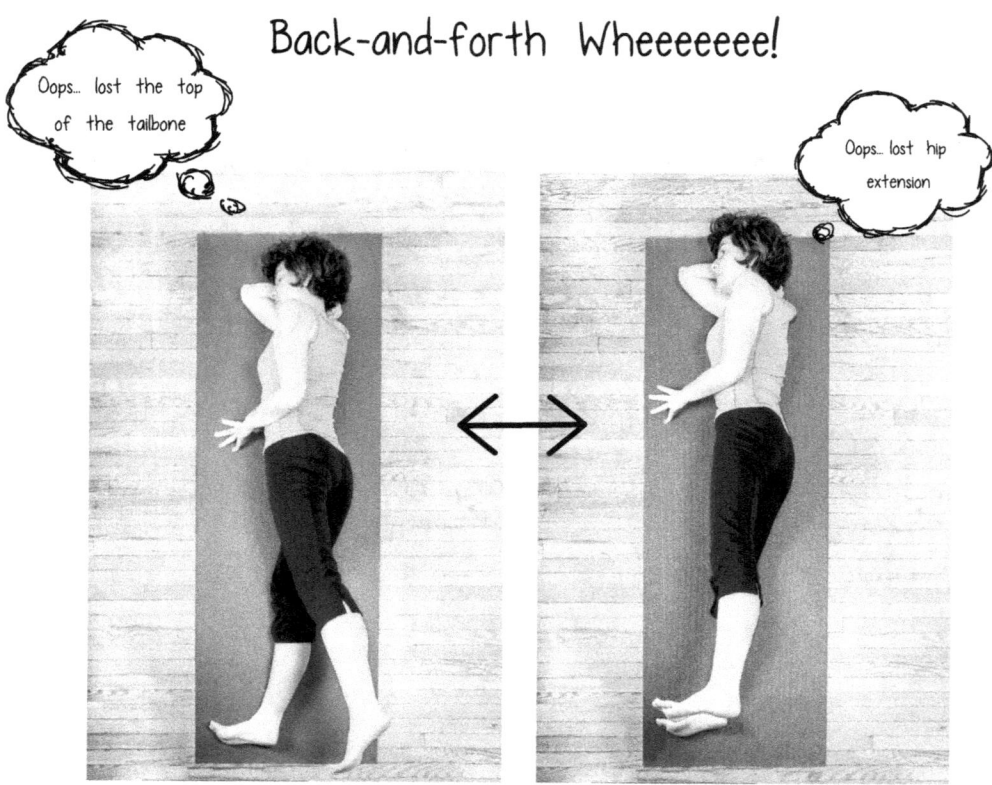

No worries if one drops, just find it again. Eventually you will find both at the same time.

What you will feel when you get both actions at the same time:

✓ Back of buttocks feels powerful (like a sprinter)
✓ Low back is supported/comfortable
✓ and you feel stable, strong, without vulnerability

Yes... you got it!

Note. New clients often say that they don't think of their body as powerful or haven't felt that sensation in a long time. Know that we all have power and strength, we just need to re-learn how to access this. Most clients will also laugh when they find hip extension at the same time as top-of-the-tailbone work... if you find yourself laughing... you likely have it and are surprised by the feeling.

Yes, that's it!

You are in position

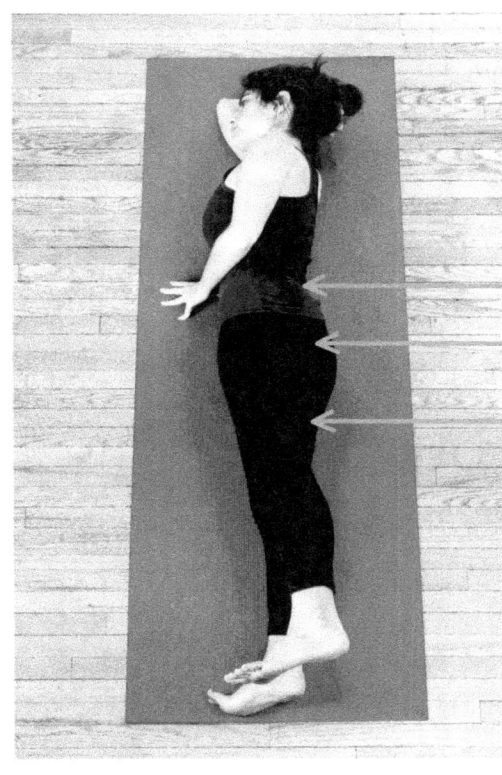

Low back feels supported ✓

Back of glutes feel powerful ✓

Back of thigh firm ✓

Flip over to your other side and repeat, combining the 2 movements, so you know how to get into position (1. Hip extension, 2. Top-of-the-tailbone work).

Doing the Leg Lifts

Try 4 - 6 leg lifts on each side

End
Position

Start
Position

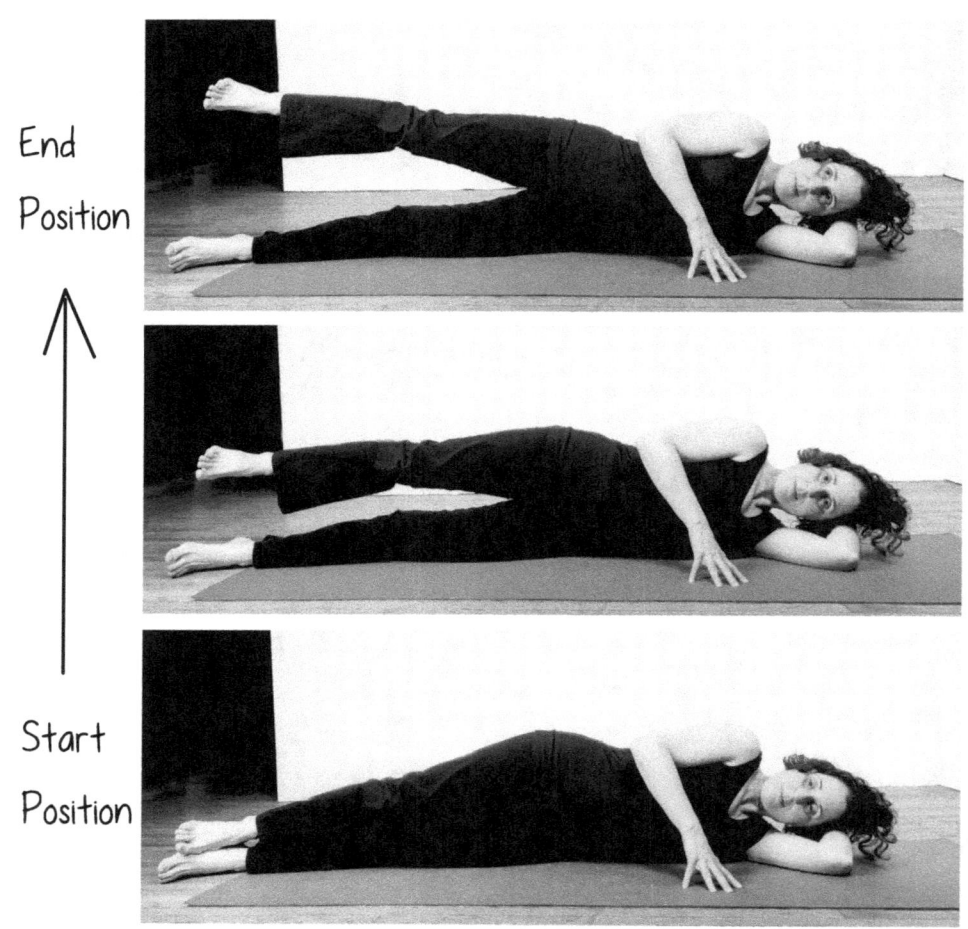

Lift and lower the leg

Do the leg lifts slowly at first, so you can maintain hip extension and a little bit of top-of-the-tailbone work throughout the leg lift up and down. If you lose it, no worries. You will be there to feel when that happens, when something has been lost, and then you will find it again during the leg lift. After you have had time to practice this, speed up the pace of the leg lifts to make it a fluid movement.

How often should I do them?

- everyday

How many should I do?

- 4 - 6 leg lifts on one side and then the other side
- then do it again

Remember this is the ideal amount. If you feel tired one day, try 1 or 2 leg lifts and see if that's good for the day. If your back is a bit sore one day, and you feel hesitant about the exercise, skip the exercise and just take 5 minutes to rest on your back, re-confirm your commitment to relieving pain, be gentle with that person who is struggling today, and know that rest is exactly what you need in this moment. You will try again tomorrow.

You may want to try:

→ Starting with the top-of-the-tailbone work and then add hip extension. Some clients have felt less discomfort in their low back or safer this way.

The thing you must watch out for is that you don't lock yourself out of doing hip extension because you are so focused on maintaining the top-of-the-tailbone work. You must allow your hip to move forward and leg to go slightly back. Your job is to resist hip extension with the littlest amount of top-of-the-tailbone work that will keep your back supported.

→ Not lifting the top leg up off the bottom leg. You still do hip extension and the top-of-the-tailbone work but no leg lift.

This is a much gentler start. You will still gain the skills needed to support your back and activate the muscles on the back of your body. This approach may be perfect for those people that have any fear of movements hurting them or are having discomfort with this exercise. There is no rush to lift the leg up and down. Let's first make sure you are comfortable and feel safe... Once you can get both movements without the leg lift, then you will be ready to lift the leg.

Main thing to know:

It's o.k. not to know how to do the leg **lift perfectly.** You will not injure yourself. Make this practice about being playful. Make it more about feeling what your body is doing... because if you can feel what your body is doing and not doing, you will know what you need to realize your full movement potential.

Just like a person starting platform diving, I wouldn't expect them to know how to do a couple of flips into the water on the first day. It takes time to build a new skill. Give yourself this time. If you do, you will get it.

CHAPTER 3

Feeling ease and comfort from our body

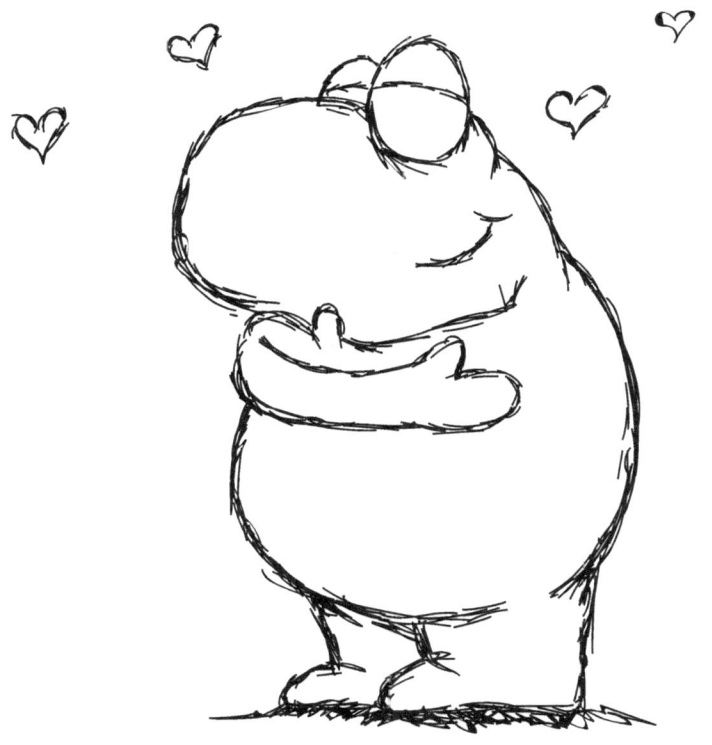

After doing 4 - 6 leg lifts on one side...

Just rest and breathe.

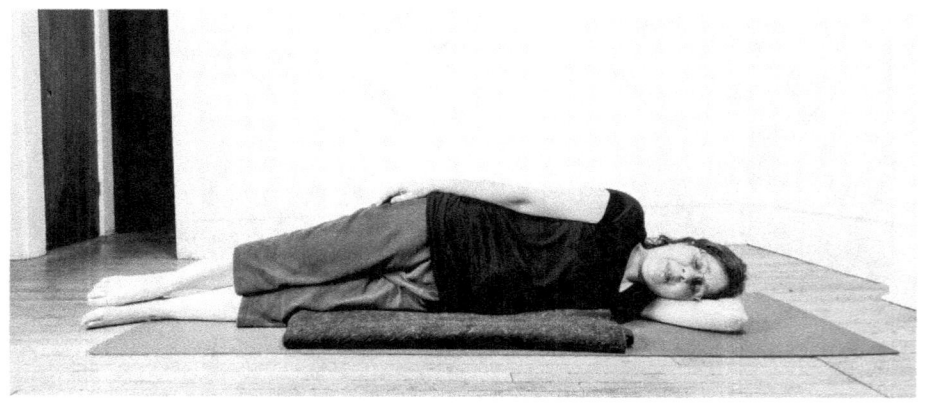

- feel how the breath begins to deepen naturally from the exercise

- take time to feel the breath at your nose

- feel your natural in-breaths... and your natural out-breaths

- feel how the body and the breath begin to warm

- and feel any good fatigue that may be there, bringing a sense of deep relaxation and weightedness

- let yourself know, "I know now, that when I feel the old pain pattern I'm not hurting myself. I'm not in danger and I don't need to protect. This is just an old protection pattern"

- rest in this deep knowing. This clarity

It is important to take time to enjoy the results of your practice.

See that the body can be a source of comfort and ease at times when you feel the whole body resting and the whole body breathing. It is also good to check-in at this point to see if any worry or pain is coming up. If there is, read pages 153 - 157 in the Summary chapter now. If your practice is bringing ease and comfort you know you are good to continue. If it is only bringing worry, tension, and discomfort; it's time to stop for today and try again tomorrow.

Note. You want to stop to feel the things that feel good because they feel good. Feeling these things will help bring a deeper relaxation response (the part of the nervous system response that says you're all good, you can chill out).

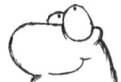

CHAPTER 4

What to do when we have a flare-up

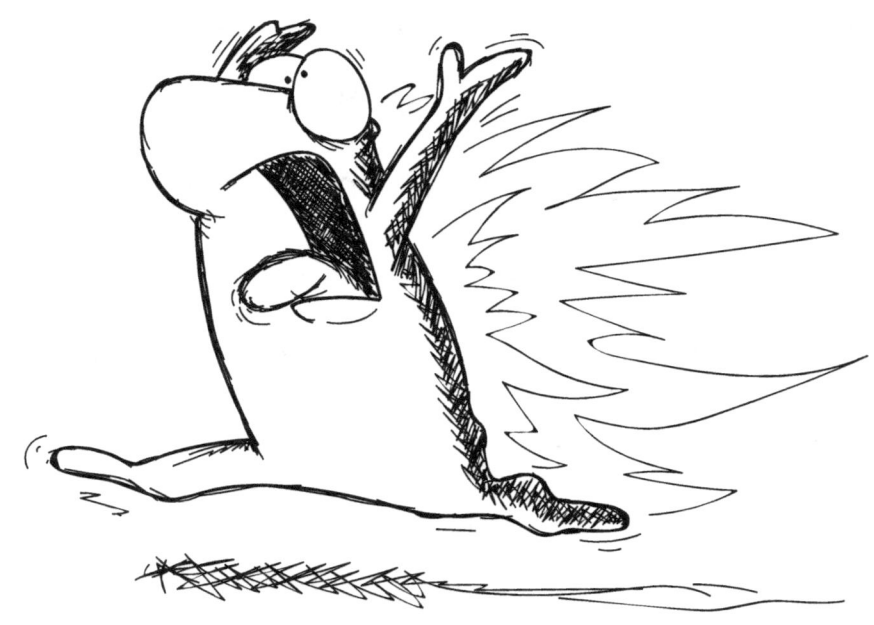

If your back flares up, know you didn't do anything wrong.

You aren't hurting yourself.

You just went past the threshold line of safety and the alarm bells went off.

Know, when you slowly introduce new movements and new challenges you never know perfectly how to stay below that threshold. I know this flare-up can be discouraging. Just give it a few days to calm down. Once it has, you will reduce the amount of leg lifts you do. There is no rush to do 4 - 6 leg lifts. Even one can be enough. You have to find the amount that does not set off the alarm bells and progress slowly from there.

You will need a little courage and support to restart each time.

Steps to try in a flare-up

Step 1:

- Take 1 - 3 days off the legs lifts until your back calms down. For these days extend kindness, support and compassion to that person who is struggling

Step 2:

- Do 1 leg lift on each side the first day you start back to see how it feels. Read pages 153 - 157.

Step 3:

- If you don't flare the next day from doing 1 leg lift, and you feel ready, do 2 leg lifts on each side this day. Each day adding 1 more until you reach 4 - 6, and only if you feel safe to do so. Read pages 153 - 157.

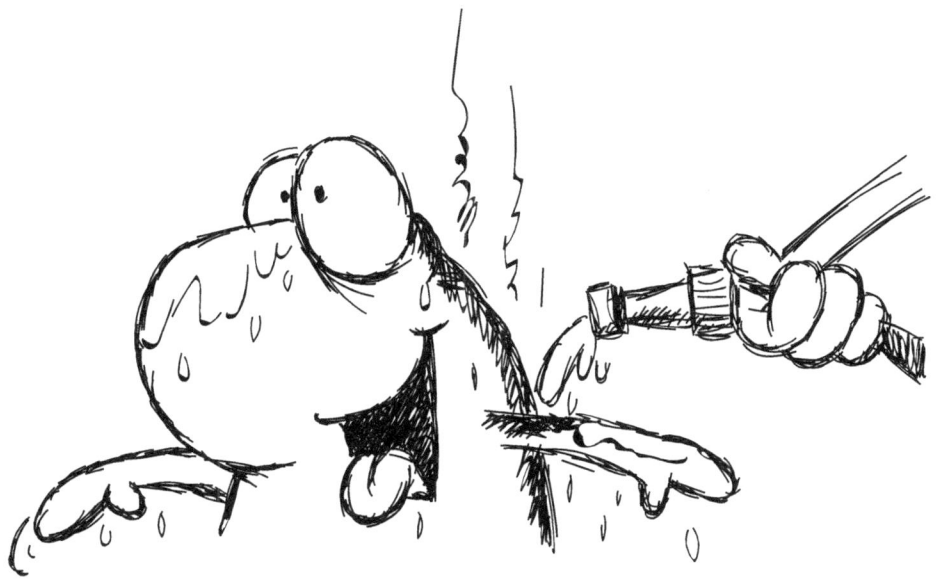

SUMMARY

What to do this week

THIS WEEK

Read through each day:

I know now...

- my old belief was: Pain = damage, injury, "something's wrong" (And this may still be present... and that's o.k.)

- my old belief was: Damage always = pain

- my new understanding is: Pain does not always = damage, injury, "something's wrong" and Damage does not always = pain, especially with chronic pain

- that I do not have an injury that needs fixing, if a recent diagnosis of something like a broken bone or dislocated hip wasn't found

- that with chronic pain I can have "damage" or degeneration and the body can be very capable and without constant pain

Continued...

I know now...

- when I feel the old pain pattern, I am not hurting myself

- bad posture, tight, or weak muscles are not the cause of my chronic pain

- when I feel the old pain pattern, its not because I did something the wrong way

- the reason I have good days is not because I have become stronger, more flexible, and now have better alignment

- the structure of my back is not the reason for my pain

- the reason I keep having back pain is because I have a sensitized nervous system

- there is no reason why I cannot make a full recovery from chronic pain and get back to the activities I love

THIS WEEK

Every time pain or worry (that something bad is going to happen) comes up, stop and ask:

1. Am I in danger of getting an actual injury right now?

(like a broken bone or dislocated hip)

Yes - stop activity

See a doctor. Let yourself know that to the best of your ability you will take yourself out of harm's way. You can trust yourself to do this.

No - proceed to the next question, but first go through the following...

If there is no feeling like a bone is going to break or a hip is going to dislocate right now, I know now that it's not true that I am in danger of an injury. This is just an old pain pattern playing. I've felt this before. And it's not true anymore.

$\rightarrow$

Note 1. Thinking that something bad is going to happen now, or later on, is not the same as being in danger of an actual injury. This is a worry cycle.

Note 2. Flare-ups (same back pain repeating itself or can't move patterns cycling every couple of months or yearly, and no injury was found on the recent physio assessment) are not actual injuries. This is the sensitivity cycle where we have passed that threshold where we think we are safe and have gone into high alert again. We think we are in danger and we need to protect. This feeling of something is wrong can be subconscious.

2. Am I too worried to continue this activity?

Yes - stop activity

Let yourself know that you will not put yourself in a situation where there is too much worry. (For example: worry about the tension you are experiencing, the worry that happens when you feel weak, or the worry that happens when you think you did something the wrong way... all of which makes you think you are going to hurt yourself). You will stop the activity and extend support, kindness, and compassion to that person who is struggling with worry right now. You will try again tomorrow when the perceived danger is not as high.

No - proceed with activity

This is where there may be a bit of worry still around, but you know theoretically or actually you are not in danger of an injury. Staying in the activity will not be overwhelming with worry.

THIS WEEK

Once a day, do the side leg lifts

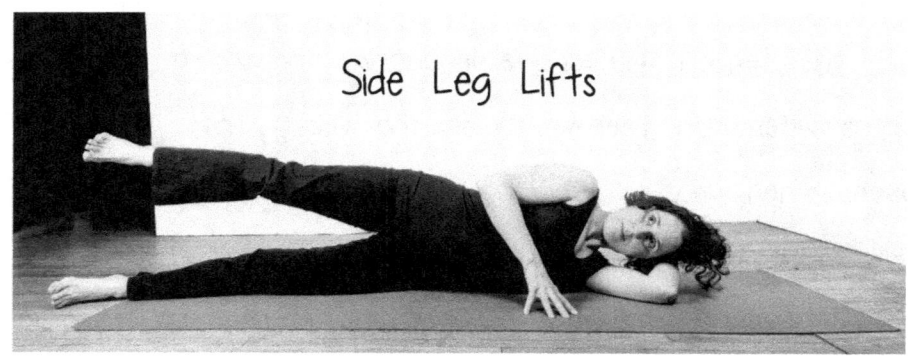

Side Leg Lifts

How many should I do?

- 4 - 6 leg lifts on one side and then repeat on the other side
- then do it again

Next Week

You will...

- add 1 mental training exercise
- add 1 physical training exercise
- do a brief review of Week 1

If you need more time to master Week 1's training, please take an extra week to do so before proceeding to Week 2. My clients' number 1 reason for not doing the training is because they don't feel confident they know how (first they say it is because they are lazy, but with a little discussion it's actually confidence). This is normal when learning a new skill. Allow your practice to be about playfulness (rather than right or wrong).

Remember, you will not hurt yourself if you do the exercises "wrong". Take your time. You will get it. You will usually underestimate how much you know or how much you can feel. If you slow things down, you will get it.

Happy Training!

Supplement

Different ways to set up the exercise for comfort

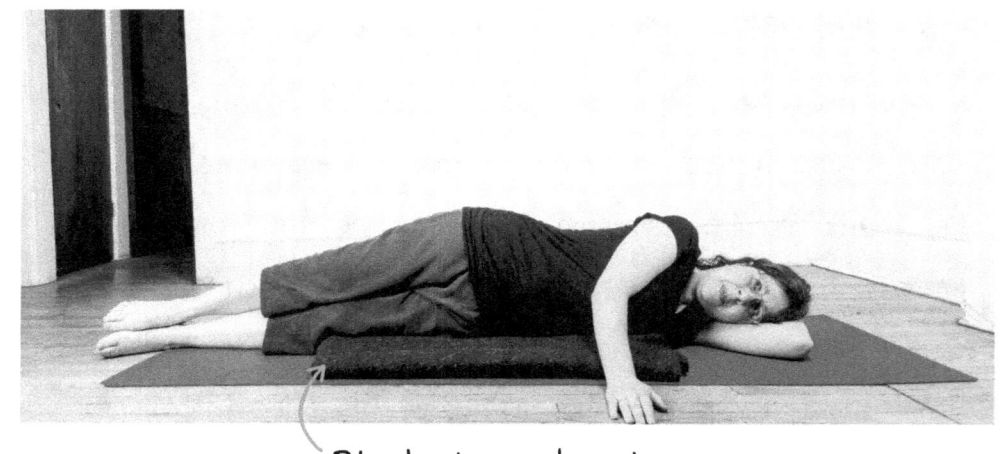

Blanket under hip

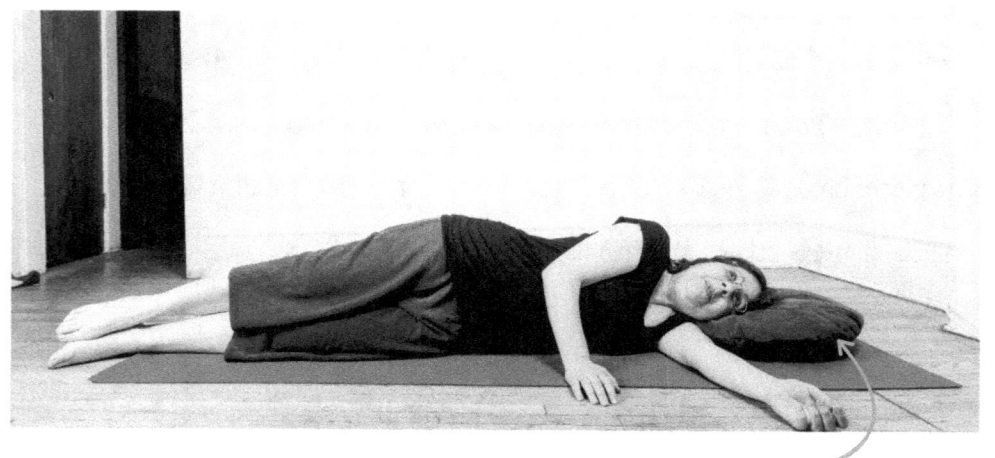

Pillow for head

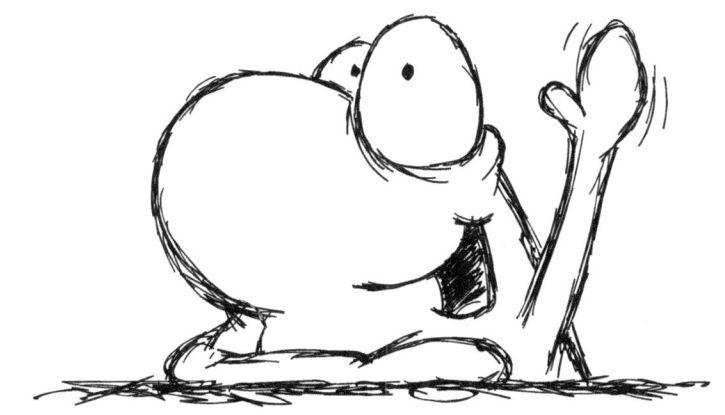

"See you next week in the next book!"

Acknowledgements

Thank you to my family for their support and love... always encouraging me to follow my dreams and heart. I am forever grateful. I love you.

Thank you to my teachers and mentors for their teachings and support... always inspiring me with new ways of learning, helping, and being. I am forever grateful. I love you.

Thank you to Katina Watson, Frances Brooks, and Angela Calderone for modeling the exercises in this series of books. I am forever grateful. I love you.

Thank you to my yoga and mindfulness communities for meeting each week with the intention of continuous learning and being in presence. My heart always looks forward to it. I am forever grateful. I love you.

Thank you to Risa Scher and Vanessa Guillen for editing this

Acknowledgements Cont.

series of books. Thank you to Chris MacLean and Maggie Bergeron for providing feedback to improve this series of books. I am forever grateful. I love you.

Thank you to all my friends for your support and laughter. Always look forward to our time together. I am forever grateful. I love you.

And thank you to all of the musicians, comedians, writers, actors, and creative people who inspire my work each day. Without this accompaniment each day I don't think these books would have been written. I am forever grateful. I love you.

About the Author

Rachel Donen was born in the Canadian prairies of Saskatoon. As a teenager, she suffered 3 major car accidents where her car was rear ended. These would be her first experiences with chronic pain.

Because of this experience Rachel knew that she wanted to help those suffering with pain so she started her physical rehabilitation training, applying to the College of Kinesiology in 1998.

During her first year of university her brother intro-duced her to the mindfulness/awareness teachings of Krishnamurti. At this time, Rachel didn't know exactly how, but she felt this work would be of great benefit to those with chronic pain. And was eager to research if any treatments for chronic pain included such ideas.

She found a handful of studies showing how cognitive-behavioural-therapy, mindfulness, and yoga had helped reduce chronic pain, anxiety, and depression. Notably, the work of researcher and clinician, Jon Kabat-Zinn. His initial mindfulness research, in an area that was at the time in its infancy, laid the groundwork for Rachel to further contribute to this field.

With the guidance of her supervisor, Kent Kowalski, Rachel's undergraduate research focused on chronic pain rehabilitation and the use/access to cognitive-behavioural therapy. Her Master's thesis provided insight into what mindfulness looked like in response to a field that was struggling to define it. Here, Rachel developed her first mindfulness program with feedback from leaders in the field, including Jon Kabat-Zinn (Mindfulness based Stress Reduction), Mark Lee (Krishnamurti Foundation of America) and Patricia Dewar (her yoga mentor).

About the Author Cont.

During this time Rachel completed a 3-year yoga teacher training program with head teachers, Patricia Dewar (Yoga Central, Saskatoon) and Mary Lou Weprin (The Yoga Room, Berkeley CA). Their mindfulness teachings of observation and playfulness through movement in yoga postures were vital in Rachel's initial direct experience of awareness. Rachel also trained with yoga teachers, Donald Moyer, Gay White, Lynne Minton, and Father Joe Pereira. (During this time Rachel developed chronic low back and knee pain.)

In 2009, Rachel moved to Toronto and opened, "Alignment Yoga" which has since become, "ALIGN physical rehab". She switched from a yoga class business to one that treated chronic pain and injury as she found almost all of her students suffering in this way... and because this was always a passion of hers.

Rachel furthered her studies in mindfulness, with 5 years

of meditation and awareness training with Buddhist nun Ani Jamyang Donma and awareness teacher Christopher Aslan. Rachel also trained with Jack Kornfield and studied the works of Cheri Huber, Debbie Ford, Don Miguel Ruiz, and Marshall Rosenberg.

Rachel gained knowledge in neuroscience. In 2013, she was introduced to neuroscience research explaining pain, by physiotherapist and chiropractor Greg Lehman. Notably, the works of Lorimer Mosely and David Butler guided her understanding of the nervous system in relation to chronic pain. When Rachel integrated her knowledge and direct experience of mindfulness, neuroscience, kinesiology, and yoga with her clients' stories of chronic pain, she saw the need for a formal program to help people recover from chronic pain. She developed these books so that others have a direct path to recovering from chronic pain.

About the Author Cont.

Rachel's books provide a new approach to chronic pain recovery. Just like her teachers helped guide her recovery from chronic pain and provided insight into her full potential, her wishes are that these books may be of help to all of those people still in pain. Rachel is forever grateful for these teachings.

Work with Rachel

- On-line
- In Person
- By Phone

Rachel conducts private sessions on how to recover from chronic pain. For those that would like one-on-one attention and guidance in addition to her books. To book with Rachel go to:

www.alignphysicalrehab.com for more information

Books also by Rachel:

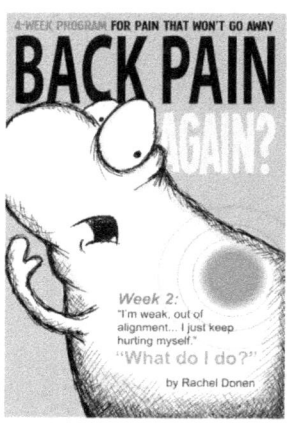

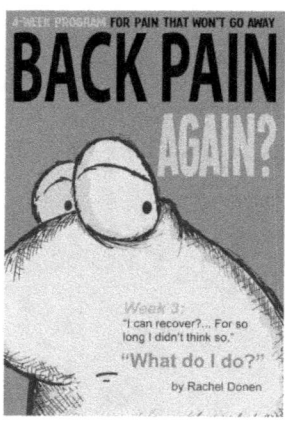

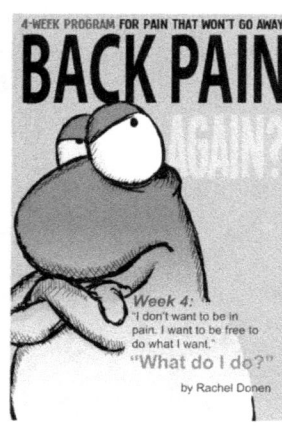

www.ingramcontent.com/pod-product-compliance
Lightning Source LLC
Chambersburg PA
CBHW072046280526
45788CB00006B/2197